From ME to

FROM ME TO Me
A Journey of Healing, Reiki and Rediscovering Myself

C 2025 Diane Carole
All rights reserved

No part of this book may be reproduced, stored in a retrieval system, or transmitted in any form or by any means - electronic, mechanical, photocopying, recording, or otherwise - without prior written permission of the author, except in the case of brief quotations used in reviews or articles.

This is a work of nonfiction.

ISBN:

Cover design C 2025 Diane Carole

Published by Amazon KDP
Printed in United Kingdom

DISCLAIMER

The experiences and advice shared in this memoir reflect the personal journey of the author and are provided for informational purposes only. They are not intended to replace professional medical advice, diagnosis or treatment. Always seek the guidance of your doctor or other qualified health provider with any questions you may have regarding diet, exercise or your health condition. Never disregard professional medical advice or delay in seeking it because of something you may have read in this book. Your health is unique to you, and what works for one person may not be appropriate for another.

TABLE OF CONTENTS

Acknowledgements
Foreword

1. M.E.
    Finding Light in the Shadows - *Affirmations/Mantras*
    Empowering Healing Suggestions
    Journaling Reflection Questions
    Poem - The First Step

2. *Finding Reiki*
    Opening to the Healing Light - *Affirmations/Mantras*
    Empowering Healing Suggestions
    Journaling Reflection Questions
    Poem - The Hands Remember

3. *Spiritual Growth*
    Awakening the Inner Light - *Affirmations/Mantra*
    Empowering Healing Suggestions
    Journaling/Reflection Questions
    Poem - Becoming

4. *The Birth of Tranquility*
    Stepping Into The Dream - *Affirmations/Mantras*
    Empowering Healing Suggestions
    Journaling/Reflection Questions
    Poem - The Threshold

5. *Tranquility Holistic Centre*
    Expanding Into Possibility - *Affirmations/Mantras*
    Empowering Healing Suggestions
    Journaling Reflection Questions
    Poem - The Garden You Planted

6. *The Divorce*
   Finding Myself In The Quiet - Affirmations/Mantras
                                  Empowering Healing Suggestions
                                  Journaling Reflection Questions
                                  Poem - The Quiet That Heals

7. *The Travels*
   The Courage To Begin Again - Affirmations/Mantras
                                  Empowering Healing Suggestions
                                  Journaling Reflection Questions
                                  Poem - The Phoenix Within

8. *Homeless*
   Unshakeable Spirit - Affirmations/Mantras
                             Empowering Healing Suggestions
                             Journaling Reflection Questions
                             Poem - The Road Still Rises

9. *The Discovery*
   Standing In My Strength - Affirmations/Mantras
                                Empowering Healing Suggestions
                                Journaling Reflection Questions
                                Poem - I See Her Now

10. *The Lessons in Finding ME*
    Living As The Whole Self - Affirmations/Mantras
                                   Empowering Healing Suggestions
                                   Journaling Reflection Questions
                                   Poem - Home At Last

ACKNOWLEDGEMENTS

"Through the stillness of my body,
I learned the language of my soul.
Through the light in my hands,
I found my way home to me."

To everyone who has been part of my life in anyway - thank you. Whether you have brought joy, challenge, love or lessons, each of you has helped shape the person I am today. I now see that every experience, every circumstance, has been a step on my path of healing and self-discovery.

And to you, the reader - by holding this book in your hands, you've now become part of my journey too.
For that, I am truly grateful.

DEDICATION

For everyone walking the path of healing, self-discovery, and self-love - may you find hope in the pages ahead, strength in your own story, and the courage to keep going, even on the hardest days.

And for the version of me who never gave up - this is for you.

FOREWORD

The reason I wish to share my story is in the hope that it reaches anyone who is wanting to grow on the path of self discovery, self growth, self belief and self love and hope that it helps them in some way.

I'm going to start my story from the age of 28, (1998), when my whole world was turned upside down and shaken to the core, I became very unwell, it took a long time to get a diagnosis of what was wrong with me. The diagnosis was M.E. (Myalgic Encephalomyelitis) also known as CFS (Chronic Fatigue Syndrome) and this changed my life, leading me in a totally different direction of what I had planned and how I thought my life would turn out. Its been extremely tough over the years with many highs and lows but what has transpired over this time has been a massive learning curve in which I have learned some very valuable tools, this in turn has lead me to overhaul my lifestyle and how I now look at this precious gift of life. This is what I'll be sharing with you throughout the book. The reason I have decided to write this book now, is that this year, 2023, I have finally found ME, after so many changes, I feel strong, mentally, physically, emotionally and spiritually. I am stepping into my authentic self. I am fully embracing life, each and every day. A lot has changed this year and I have come to the realisation that I now know who I am, what I want, what's important to me and what makes me happy. I am far from perfect but each day I strive to be the best version of myself and live life to the best of my ability, creating as many memories as I can and living in the moment and as I do this I continue to grow on my path of self discovery, self growth, self belief and self love. I know for certain I still have so much to learn.

Writing this book, which stems over the last 25 years has been very healing for me and made me realise how much I have went through and how this path, as difficult as it has been over the years it has changed me in so many ways. The path to self discovery, self growth, self belief and self love is not easy for anyone but I do believe to find ourselves we have to look within and continue to learn from the lessons that life teaches us.

If reading this story can help even one person in some way then that will make me happy.

CHAPTER ONE - DIAGNOSIS OF M.E.

This year 1998, was very memorable for me. I got married that year and shortly after I began getting unwell. This got progressively worse over time, most days I could not get out of bed and in the year, 2000, I was finally diagnosed with M.E.

My wedding day was a happy event and everything went perfectly. By the end of the evening my mouth felt a bit achy but I put it down to all the smiling and talking I'd done all day. We stayed to the end of the night then travelled back to our home in Helensburgh, where we had our cases all packed and ready for our trip to the airport with a friend, a couple of hours later. If I remember right, it was around 4.00 a.m. when we got to the airport to fly out to Cyprus for our honeymoon. My mouth and jaw were still achy, but I tried not to think about it too much.

The pain got worse on the plane. I was in agony, then one side of my face, my nose, chin and forehead all became very swollen. By the time we landed, my face was all distorted and I was in so much pain. We checked into the hotel, then went to the hospital. I got antibiotics and thankfully they did begin to work pretty quickly. When we flew home a week later, my face had returned to normal size, and I looked more like myself again, but I still had some pain in my mouth.

I quickly got booked into the dentist when I got home. I got more antibiotics, as I had an abscess in my gums. The pain continued and nothing seemed to ease it. I kept having different work done to my teeth, even having one of my molars removed but the pain continued and over the next few months I got lots more antibiotics. Eventually I got referred to a professor in Glasgow, as I was now constantly in pain and feeling unwell.

After doing different tests, the professor told me he needed to cut into my gums once more to investigate. He found a massive infection, going from one side of the bottom gum to the other, where my two bottom wisdom teeth had grown sideways at the back of my gums, never breaking through because there wasn't enough room in my mouth for them. This positioning had allowed an infection to build up behind them and make it difficult to find out what was wrong. I now had to get these two teeth removed - but this meant a three-day stay in hospital so they could cut into the back of my gums, break up the teeth and take them out this way.

The day of the operation came, and I went to theatre and got the general anaesthetic. The next thing I remember was being in the ward. I could only open my mouth very slightly, the two sides of my mouth were all stitched up and for the next few days I could only have fluids which I had to drink through a straw. A few days later I progressed to foods, that didn't take any chewing, like mashed potatoes. Although the whole procedure was not a pleasant experience, the pain I had been experiencing for all those months was finally gone.

Going through such pain over many months had taken its toll. There was this constant tiredness and I couldn't shake it. It wasn't a normal tiredness. I felt exhausted, my body ached, I felt nauseous, and I kept losing my balance. I fought my body and kept going and going, pushing myself. All I wanted was to feel normal again. I now realise this was the wrong thing to do - but this lesson took years for me to learn. I never listened to what my body was telling me. It was telling me to rest and recover, to get myself better. Maybe you've done this too? Always soldiering on, putting others needs before your own, running yourself into exhaustion, criticising or berating yourself, being extremely hard on yourself and taking on everyone else's burdens while not listening to your own needs.

Over time, I got progressively worse and the symptoms were constant. I went from working full-time hours to part-time hours. Finally I got diagnosed with M.E. It was now the year 2000. To be honest, I was happy to finally have a diagnosis. It was so hard to not know what was wrong with me, it had been really tough. I eventually went from working part-time to being unable to work at all. I had no energy and some days I literally crawled to the bathroom or held on to the wall to get there as the dizziness and fatigue made me so unwell.

Having the diagnosis allowed me to research this condition and find out as much as I could about it. I could only do this on days I felt a little stronger, as even reading had become a struggle for me and these feelings of exhaustion, nausea, dizziness and despair continued to plague my life.

Over the months that followed, I tried everything that I heard of or read about in the hope that I would feel better. I just wanted to feel normal again and be able to live my life normally. I tried various different remedies and treatments that had worked for others. Looking back I was so impatient and so wanted an instant cure,2that I never really gave anything time to work. The body takes a while to process new things and sometimes it takes time to see results. I just seemed to jump from one thing to another in the hope that a miracle would happen and I would wake up feeling normal, back to my old self.

Nothing seemed to work and my health just continued to get worse. I very rarely ventured outdoors and my life became this vicious circle of feeling awful and living in my head. Everything suffered because of this condition. Over time, I lost friendships since I rarely had the energy to talk, let alone meet up with anyone. My home life suffered. I was no longer able to work, and found myself with no confidence or self-worth.

I got a lot of negative thoughts around this time, and I couldn't shake this feeling of hopelessness, "Why me?" I wondered. "Is this my life now?". This constant deterioration of my mind, body, soul? The only way I can describe it was a heaviness that engulfed my whole body, my whole mind, my soul itself. And I couldn't see how I was going to ever feel alright again. I felt so alone; nobody understood what I was going through. But looking back, neither did I, so how did I expect anyone else to be able to understand?

There were days when I felt a surge of energy and the excitement that would bring. Just feeling semi-normal again was immense and that would have me doing all the jobs around the house that needed to be done or going for a little walk. Just having some energy to do these things gave me hope but, inevitably, a day or two later I would be totally exhausted again and this became a cycle that I found hard to break. Looking back, it sounds crazy and I can see where I went wrong on those days. But to feel that bit of energy felt so good. I had always been a very busy person, so having the energy to do even the simplest of things got me so excited that I did too much. This is a time when I should have had some balance and rested instead of over-exerting myself. I learned the hard way; this seems to be a running theme during my life - never taking the easy path.

In 2001, I found out that I was pregnant. The first couple of months were very difficult but as the pregnancy grew I began to feel a little bit better and my energy began to grow too, I was still unwell, some days were better than others, but there was a definite shift. In 2002, I gave birth to a beautiful baby boy. He was 3 weeks early and had to be delivered by caesarian section, but he was healthy and I was happy, and his two older sisters were delighted with his arrival.

The first few weeks after the birth were difficult and he appeared to have day and night confused. Even though I was also recovering from the C-section I was managing alright and would try and get a nap while he was sleeping. Eventually, I was able to get out and walk with the pram, and things were improving, although I 5did have to be careful of balancing how much I was doing and the symptoms of M.E., as they did get worse if I overdid things.

Even though I was happy with the new addition to our family, and my son was a bundle of joy, my self-confidence was at an all-time low and I struggled to mix or chat with anyone I didn't know. We were living in a town where, I didn't know anyone; this made it even easier for me to isolate myself from others, but it did nothing for my self-esteem. I had always suffered from shyness, so it wasn't easy for me to meet other parents of young children and babies.

I tried to figure out, how I got M.E., I wondered if taking lots of antibiotics and having more than one general anaesthetic in the last few years had affected my immune system. Or was it from chicken pox had got in 1995? Was it because some very stressful events I had had in previous years? Was it because at the time of becoming ill I was working full-time, converting a loft extension and decorating my new home, as well as bringing up a young family and planning a wedding.

I realise now that it could've been any of these factors, or an accumulation of them, or something else completely different. But what I have discovered over the last 25 years is you have to have balance in your life and look after yourself mind, body and soul.

I have learnt that what we consume in our body has such a major impact on how our body works. We have to find what works for us, what makes us feel good, and what disagrees with us. And we need to put into practise eating what makes us feel good. We must keep our bodies hydrated, they are around 66% water, although this figure can vary, so we should keep this at a healthy balance as we lose water through sweating, urinating, crying and breathing. Drinking lots of water keeps our body balanced at the level it requires.

Exercise is also important. We need to stretch our bodies, exercise regularly, and be outdoors. Walking outdoors is so healing for the body, it keeps us fit and healthy.

What goes on in our minds is another big factor. Thinking about the past or worrying about the future has a big impact on our body. We must try and live for the now, we must be mindful of our thoughts. Stress is very damaging to us. What I have found out over time is if I allow myself to get stressed, my body begins again to get all the M.E. symptoms very quickly. After years of working with others who have M.E. or other autoimmune illness, I have also noticed something very interesting; they have all been empathetic people who take on others' problems and tend to hold on to them. As empathetic people, we are not taught how to protest our energies, but I feel it is important to learn how to do this.

Throughout this book I will share all the things I did to get better and what has worked for me. Although I keep feeling better and I live life to the full, M.E. never goes away. I have learnt how to manage it, but if I allow my body to get out of balance it doesn't take long for the symptoms to return. I'm only human and this does happen, especially if I allow myself to get stressed in anyway. But I quickly use the tools I have learned and put them into, stricter practise, allowing me to feel well again. Changing my lifestyle, mind, body and soul has allowed me to live normally.

The next chapter tells of a major turning point in my life: when I discovered Reiki, or did it discover me? As the saying goes, the teacher always appears when the student is ready.

FINDING LIGHT IN THE SHADOWS

AFFIRMATIONS/MANTRAS

- I am more than my diagnosis.
- My body is listening, and it knows how to heal.
- Every breath I take is a step toward renewal.
- I honour my body's wisdom
- I choose to see hope, even in uncertainty.

EMPOWERING HEALING SUGGESTIONS/TECHNIQUES

1. GENTLE REST WITHOUT GUILT - Give yourself permission to rest fully without labelling it as "laziness" or "wasting time." Rest is medicine.
2. BODY SCAN MEDITATION - Spend 5 minutes noticing each part of your body and sending it gratitude.
3. SOOTHING BREATHWORK - Inhale for 4 counts, exhale for 6 counts, repeating for 5 minutes to calm the nervous system.
4. NATURE CONNECTION - Sit outside or near an open window daily, feeling the sun or breeze on your skin.
5. MINI GRATITUDE RITUAL - Each night, write down 3 small moments of comfort or peace from your day.

JOURNALING REFLECTION QUESTIONS

- When I first received my diagnosis, what thoughts or fears came up for me?

- How has my relationship with my body changed since becoming unwell?

- What small comforts or daily rituals bring me peace right now?

- How do I define "healing" in this season of my life?

- If my body could speak, what might it want me to know?

- Additional reflection or memories that surface.

THE FIRST STEP

Even in the stillness,
Your spirit breathes -
Quietly, steadily,
Keeping the flame alive.

Though the world has slowed,
You are not broken.
You are the quiet seed beneath the soil,
Resting before the bloom.

The earth holds you,
The seasons wait for you,
And the sun will find you again.

The winds will carry your name,
Through branches and across oceans,
Reminding you that you are part of something vast.

Every moment of rest,
Is a whisper of renewal.
Every gentle breath
Is a step toward the horizon.

This is not the end -
This is the scared beginning.
You are walking a path
That will bring you home to yourself.

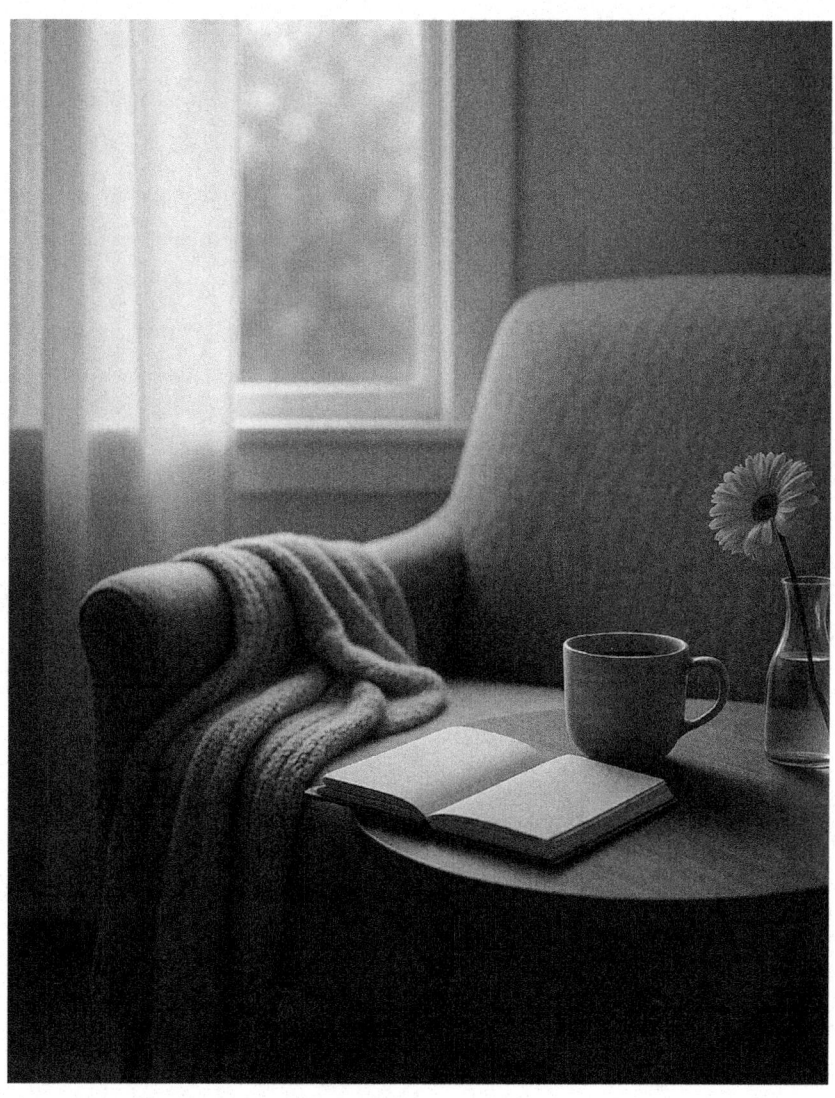

Finding Light in the Shadows

CHAPTER TWO - FINDING REIKI

I didn't realise at the time, but learning Reiki was such a defining moment for me - definitely a spiritual awakening. It changed my life in so many ways, not like a big bolt from the sky but gradually change over time. I am a completely different person now to who I was all those years ago. I do believe I have opened up to being the authentic me. After all the years of feeling that I didn't fit it. I don't want to fit in anymore. I am happy to be different, I am happy to be me and to know who I am, what I like and what I want to do and achieve. And although there will certainly be lots more twists and turns as I continue to learn and grow. I know I am who I am who I was supposed to be.

How I discovered Reiki was pretty remarkable too. What has happened over the years since, and from listening to stories of how it found other people as well. I believe that Reiki finds you - and always at the right time. Reiki is all to do with the energies. It works on the mental, emotional, physical and spiritual aspects of you and begins to heal these aspects, changing everything from the inside out and knowing exactly what your body needs at the time of using or receiving it. Reiki is channelled through us and we don't control it in any way; it flows and always flows for the greater and highest good. We don't know everything about energies, but having an understanding of them can be life-changing, if you allow it. We are energetic beings, so I believe it can only be good for us to understand a little bit about ourselves and how energy works.

By December 2003, I was still suffering from M.E., I was certainly better than I had been, and I was now able to get through the day without going for a sleep, but there was no way that I was able to work to do anything strenuous at this point in my life. The cycle of "good" and "bad" days remained. For Christmas, my parents gave me a gift voucher for a Beauty Salon that wasn't too far from where I lived. I looked through the list of available treatments and booked myself in for a Reiki treatment. I had no idea what Reiki was, but felt drawn to choose this.

The day I went for the treatment, I lay on the massage bed and the therapist began the treatment by gently placing her hands on me. I could feel this strong heat coming from her hands, I can't quite remember how long we were in the treatment before my body starting reacting to the energy, but it began pulsating very visibly,. Even though my body was moving around a lot, I wasn't frightened at this time; in fact I felt quite calm and my intuition was telling me everything was alright. The therapist had never seen anything like this before and instinctively gave me the number of her Reiki teacher, saying I should give her a call.

I did just that. I'm not sure how it happened , but I found myself signed up to do the Reiki One course on 2nd February 2004. The date came and I was extremely nervous. I was nervous about driving there, as it was 25 miles away and I had rarely driven for years now and certainly not that distance. I was nervous because I didn't really know what I was getting into. I didn't really understand what Reiki was . And I was nervous because I had to go into a room full of people I didn't know and communicate and learn with them.

Despite my nerves, everything went well. I didn't have to worry about being there with others as I ended up in the class by myself. The teacher had actually rescheduled the class, but she had only realised that morning that she had forgotten to phone me. I do believe that the energies were at work and I was supposed to be at that class by myself.

During the class, the teacher, introduced me to Reiki, attuned me to Reiki One and taught me how to do a self-treatment and, a treatment on others. Later on in the day, she asked if I would like a tarot card reading and I happily had a reading done. A couple of things she said during the reading have always stayed with me; the first was she told me that I was a natural healer and would use the Reiki to help myself and others; the second thing she said that sticks in my mind was that I should be reading tarot cards like her, or reading tea leaves like my gran did as it ran in my family. I had no idea that Gran did this and I asked my dad when I got home. He confirmed that she did read tea leaves for others.

Although at the time I couldn't see how this could happen, it has. I used Reiki to heal myself. I now use it to help others and I teach Reiki classes. I also read tarot cards for others.

Before I left that day, I signed up to do the Reiki Two class, which was being held on 4th April 2004. In the meantime, I started doing a 21-day self-healing that was part of Reiki One, I did it religiously every day. My routine was to do it in my bed before going to sleep. I loved it. I loved the way it made me feel and I knew it was helping me; it was working on my body mentally, emotionally, physically and spiritually and at a gentle pace that my body could cope with.

I was still nervous going to the Reiki Two class, but not as much as I'd felt with Reiki One. There were five others in the class, it went well, and we were all attuned to the Reiki Two level. I love the feeling of an attunement; there is something special about it. Being attuned to Reiki 2 allowed me to be a practitioner. This wouldn't happen immediately for me, as there was still a lot of healing my body required. After the class, I did my 21-day self-healing everyday and continued using it as much as I could after that. In fact, this is what I still do to this day. I love using Reiki, it is my absolute passion.

I have learned so much about Reiki over the years and it never fails to amaze me. I walked into the first class having no idea what it was about, but over the years it has taught me so much and it has helped me heal in so many ways. The process seemed slow to me at first, but when I look back at everything, it was all in divine timing. To heal I also had to learn a lot of lessons and let go of a lot of fear and anger that I held onto.

I would like to share a little about Reiki and give you my interpretation of how energy works in the hope that it helps you understand it a little better.

Reiki was discovered in Japan in the late 19th century by Dr Usui. Rei (pronounced "ray") means universal and Ki(pronounced "key)" means life energy. Ki flows through our energy pathways - our chakras and meridians - and, around us in a field of energy called the aura. This flow of Ki keeps the body balanced and healthy; when the flow is blocked, the body is unbalanced and stress, stress-related illnesses and depression are then allowed to thrive. Reiki works on balancing the body and unblocking the body's own ability to heal itself and relieve aches and pains, muscle strain, stress, fear, depression, and feelings of anger and sadness. It brings an overall feeling of wellbeing to the recipient. It is also beneficial as a preventive treatment to help maintain good health.

I have been using the word energy a lot, but what is energy? Energy is life. It is the invisible force that animates the human body and, permeates everything in the natural world, including animals, plants, trees and rocks, as well as the Earth, Sun, Moon and stars. Throughout the course of history, cultures worldwide have acknowledged the existence of a universal energy force flowing through everything in the world, including the human body. Today, many people refer to it as "life force". Invisible like the air we breathe, the life force is balanced and allowed to flow freely. When it is blocked or unbalanced, it leads to disturbances that will eventually manifest as "dis-ease" or a state of disharmony in the natural order. Energy healing is all about finding ways to strengthen, balance and free up this energy.

We all have storage centres in our bodies that store energy and energy patterns. These are called chakras. We can have energy patterns stored from events that, happened yesterday or many years ago. Some of these patterns will be happy memories, and some of them will be unpleasant and painful memories. Sometimes we stash these memories away deep in, some recess in our chakras and in our auras and try to forget about them, but they don't really go away. Dis-ease is a manifestation of unbalanced energy; healing then is a way of balancing energy.

The human aura, also known as the spiritual aura, is energy emanating from the spinal column. The energy comes from the combination of body, soul and mind working together in a person. Everything that you are, that you have done, and even that you could do is beamed out of your spiritual force field. Auras look like the wavering energy field around the Sun. They are constantly shifting in size, shape and colouring, in perfect unison with the person's thoughts and emotions.

Meridians of the body affect every organ and physiological system inside us. They are invisible to the human eye, yet without them we would not sustain life. In the same way that arteries carry blood, meridians carry energy. Meridians are our "energy bloodstreams"; they bring vitality and balance; remove energy blockages, stagnations and imbalances; adjust metabolism; and determine the speed and form of cellular change. Their flow is as critical as the flow of blood - your life and health depend on both. Meridians of the body affect all major systems, including : the immune, nervous, endocrine, circulatory, respiratory, digestive, skeletal, muscular and lymphatic systems. If a meridian's energy is obstructed or unregulated, the system it feeds on is jeopardised and disease results.

Here are some important facts about Reiki to keep in mind:

- It channels universal life energy to promote, relaxation and a feeling of wellbeing.
- It is safe and simple.
- It can benefit anyone regardless of background, education, religious beliefs or age.
- It is complementary to conventional medicine.
- It uses hands with a gentle touch on a fully clothed body.
- It produces feelings of peace and harmony.
- It promotes the healing of injuries.
- It helps support other complementary therapies.
- It is non-invasive.
- It can be used to treat plants and animals, as well as people.
- It is not a religion, nor does it contradict any religious beliefs.

- It charges the body with positive energy, thus allowing the life force to flow in a healthy and natural way.

People may feel various sensations when giving or receiving Reiki. Some people may feel nothing or little at all, but be assured Reiki is still working. Here is a list of experiences which are quite common during a Reiki treatment : sensations of heat or cold, gentle tingling, rippling sensations, inner vibration, involuntary movements, seeing beautiful colours, past life flashes, dreams or visions and memory flashes. Quite often, people fall asleep.

I believe that if you allow Reiki to do its work, you will find it a life-changing experience.

What I found through learning about Reiki was how important it is for us to protect our energies. I do feel, especially if we are empathetic, that we take on others' energies. For example, if you are in the company of someone who constantly moans or speaks negatively, you may feel totally drained afterwards. Even more than that, you may actually hold onto that energy within your chakras, aura and meridians. The techniques I use to prevent this happening are protection, cleansing and grounding. There are several ways to do this, and I will give examples of what I do. Doing this daily will make a big difference to you. It's worth learning these practises and making them a habit; they don't take long to do but will benefit you in several ways.

PROTECTION TECHNIQUE

Using the protection technique will protect you from negative energies or energies from a lower vibration and it will help keep your energy balanced. How I protect my energies is by closing my eyes, taking three deep breaths, and with a prayer of intent - asking for a bubble of protection to surround me. I imagine this beautiful clear bubble surrounding my whole body. (You could make it any colour, even sparkly if that's what you prefer.) I then silently acknowledge my gratitude by saying "thank you" three times.

CLEANSING TECHNIQUE

Using the cleansing technique will allow you to release impurities, built-up energy, negative energy, stuck energy or toxins from your body. It also disconnects your energy from others. How I cleanse my energy is again by closing my eyes, taking three deep breaths, and imagining myself standing under a beautiful waterfall and allowing the water to run down over me, clearing everything unwanted away. I watch the water flow away down a stream and then silently acknowledge my gratitude by saying "thank you" three times.

GROUNDING TECHNIQUE

Using the grounding technique strengthens your connection to universal life energy. It will increase your physical energy by expanding and connecting your aura to draw from the universal energy system. How I ground my energy is by firstly closing my eyes, taking three deep breaths, and then imagining, my body like a tree trunk, with roots spreading from the soles of my feet deep down into the earth. I feel myself strong and grounded. I then silently acknowledge my gratitude by saying "thank you" three times.

These are the methods that I use, but there are several different ways that you can do these techniques. It's all about finding what you are comfortable doing and what feels right for you. Everything is done with intent, so just intending that the techniques will assist you in looking after your energies will bring changes to you. Be aware of you energies !!

Now that I was attuned to Reiki and practising it whenever I could lots of serendipities started to occur and I was beginning to feel better than I had in years. Although I still had good and bad days, and times that my M.E. symptoms flared quite badly. I was definitely healing and opening up to a new spiritual path that was changing me in all ways.

OPENING TO THE HEALING LIGHT

AFFIRMATIONS/MANTRAS

- I am open to receive healing in all forms.
- Energy flows freely through me, restoring balance.
- I am grounded, protected and held in light.
- My hands carry the power to soothe and renew.
- I trust the wisdom go the universal energy.

EMPOWERING HEALING SUGGESTIONS/TECHNIQUES

1. DAILY ENERGY SWEEP - Visualise golden light washing down through your body, clearing any heaviness.
2. HAND-ON-HEART PAUSE - Place both hands over your heart and breathe deeply, feeling warmth and safety.
3. CLEANSING SHOWER RITUAL - Imagine the water carrying away emotional and energetic debris as it flows off your skin.
4. GROUNDING WALK - Walk barefoot on grass or soil for at least 5 minutes to anchor your energy.
5. PROTECTIVE LIGHT SHIELD - Visualise yourself surrounded by a shimmering bubble of light before entering busy or draining spaces.

JOURNALLING REFLECTION QUESTIONS

- What does "energy" mean to me, and how do I experience it?

- How do I feel after giving or receiving Reiki ?

- What is my current practise for protecting my own energy?

- In what ways has Reiki or positive energies shifted my mental or emotional state?

- How might I invite more light and healing into my daily routine?

- Additional reflection or memories that surface.

THE HANDS REMEMBER

Your hands are not empty -
They hold sunlight,
Gentle rivers,
And the quiet hum of creation.

They remember
What the mind forgets -
The ancient ways of soothing,
The unspoken language of love.

When you lay them gently, the body listens,
tired cells awaken,
The breath slows,
And the heart sighs in relief.

Through you,
Light travels
From the great beyond
To the smallest space within.

With each touch,
The world becomes softer,
The body remembers its song,
And the spirit, long in its shadow,
Steps into the language of light.

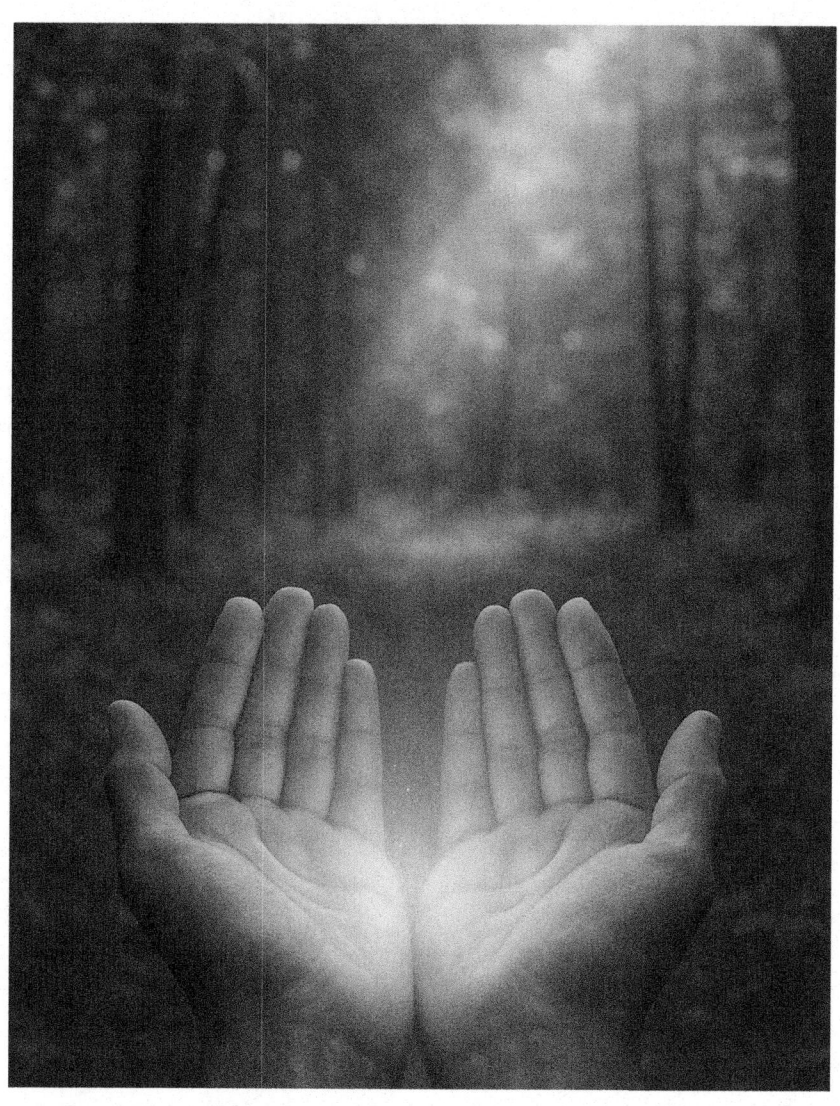

Opening to the Healing Light

CHAPTER 3 - SPIRITUAL GROWTH

Being attuned to the Reiki energies and using Reiki as a self-treatment was undoubtedly a spiritual awakening for me, even though I didn't realise this until years later. I began to feel much better than I had in years, not what I would call "normal", but there was certainly a turnaround. I could cope with a full day again, most days, and could walk further and get out and about a bit more, although I still couldn't go to busy places like the supermarket. Going there was overwhelming for me and I would feel claustrophobic. I still get like this today if somewhere is too busy. I began reading books again, something that I enjoyed doing when I was younger but hadn't done for many years.

The first book I came across that was life-changing for me was 'You Can Heal your Life" by Louise Hay. I loved this book and it made me look at things from a completely different perspective. A lot of what she said made so much sense and I found it very uplifting. I started to follow Louise's advice. At first some of the things she suggested seemed way too "out there" for me, but now, all these years later, I live my life using all these practices. It's funny just taking making one change, leads to taking the steps to the next change and continues until it feels so normal and you can't imagine not using these practises.

Reading this book did change my mindset. It also gave me a hunger to learn more about leading a more spiritual life, and I read one self-help book after another, taking everything in, making changes as much as I could. What I did find was that I would dive into lots of practises and instead of taking it slowly, or doing one thing at a time, I had to be all in. Every time I did this my body became overwhelmed and, I would become unwell again. Would I ever learn? It felt like I took two steps forward and one step backwards continuously. I've always loved learning, but I do have a tendency to become consumed with what I am learning at the time. I still do this today, it does seem to be in my nature, but I have learned to be a little easier with myself.

Around the same time I was doing all this reading, I decided to advertise that I was a Reiki practitioner. Nothing came from this, and I got no business. Although I felt disappointed at the time, I have now come to realise that I still had a long way to go to heal myself and my energies were not right at this time to become a practitioner. However, my passion for this was so great that I made the decision to start leaning other therapies, in the hope that one day I would be working again and also be able to share Reiki with others.

I decided I was going to learn massage and chose to do this at night school. To train in massage, I first had to get my qualification in anatomy and physiology, so I did this the first year that I attended night school. I could have done an extra evening learning massage at the same time, but this would have been too much for me at that time. I would do the massage course the following year. I will never forget that first class at night school, I was so nervous. My heart was pounding. I felt sick and I was so scared. But I was determined to do it.

Walking into that class for the first time was awful for me; my head was low, my shoulders were hunched, and I couldn't look at anyone, let alone have a conversation. I got through the class and continued to go every week, but I never spoke with anyone that whole year. I did pass though, and I got my qualification. The following year, I went on to learn Swedish massage. I was exactly the same that year too, and although we had to practise in pairs, I rarely said a word; I was just too nervous and shy. I did love doing the massage and when I was learning massage and getting practised on was an added bonus. I qualified in Swedish massage and continued to learn lots of different therapies over the years, all in the same way, by attending night school. I did get better at communicating and the fear lessoned and my confidence began to grow as each year went by.

In 2005, I felt fit enough to begin working part-time. I looked for a job and managed to get one fairly quickly. I ended up doing a job that was completely out of my comfort zone, but looking back I now see how it was the universe's way of making me face my fears and grow. A large DIY/home furnishings shop in the next town had just expanded and was opening a showroom selling kitchens and bathrooms. They were recruiting a lot of new staff. I applied for a position working behind the tills and managed to get an interview. The interview went well and I was delighted when I got a phone call offering me a job, although it wasn't the job I had applied for, it was a job as a salesperson, selling the kitchens and bathrooms. I accepted the job offer then got extremely worried about how I was going to do this because my confidence and self-esteem were still very low at this time.

Before beginning my new job at the showroom, I had to travel to England to do a five-day residential course to learn the role. This was definitely pushing me out of my comfort zone. There were five others doing the training with me and we would all be starting together at the showroom on opening day. The course went really well and we all bonded over the five days. This made it so much easier when we started our new roles. The atmosphere in the showroom was really good as we were now all friends.

I have to admit that I really loved that job. It gave me much more confidence - more than I had ever had - and a feeling of independence again. It is funny how things work out. Being able to work again gave me so much joy, although I still had to be careful of my limitations and there were times when I struggled with it. I was getting better at listening to my body now, although not all the time, which would leave me in my bed again. It's extremely frustrating when by nature you're a very busy person but you have to live your life with limitations. I was in the job for two years and even learnt CAD (Computer Aided Design) and began designing kitchens for customers. I enjoyed the work, but in the end left to get something with more suitable hours, when my son started school.

My next place of employment was local, and I worked at the reception desk doing reception duties, admin and accounts two days a week. My new place of employment offered job-share hours, which meant I would work two days a week and another lady, who had worked there for years, worked three days a week. These working hours suited me, as I could have the balance of working, being there for my children and managing my illness. Although I found the work alright, the lady that I job-shared with, did make things very difficult for me. I never said anything or complained about it; i just put my head down and got on with it, but it was making me ill again. I wouldn't be able to sleep on the Sunday night, worrying about going to work on the Monday.

I must add that I would never put myself in this position again. I would deal with it and not allow myself to be bullied or to be that vulnerable again - another lesson I had to learn, or was it a fear I had to face. Either way, this is another thing that I have learned as I have grown spiritually over the years. It is another tool that now sits in my toolbox. Again, the universe had a hand in this, as the skills that I learnt from this job would later help me with doing my own accounts when I became self-employed, and was running my own business. Looking back, I can see how both these jobs have helped with essential life skills that I needed to be running my own Holistic Centre. During this period of employment, I longed to be working with Reiki and the other therapies that I had learned, and I was still adding to my set of skills. I was in this job for two years before my dream came true.

At the same time as working here, I came across The Secret by Rhonda Byrne, another life-changing book for me. This book gives you the tools to manifest your desires or dream life. The thought of being able to manifest anything that I wished excited me. I wanted to put these new tools into practise, and create my own reality. I wanted to see if it would work for me. I started writing every evening in my "Manifesting diary". I would fill one page with everything that I was grateful for that day and one page with everything that I wanted to manifest. I wrote in the present tense, for example "Thank you for my successful business", or "I am grateful for all the people I can help with Reiki" . As I wrote my list each night, I imagined each thing I wished to imagine as if I already had it in my life now. I would see it in my mind's eyes. Then I would add emotion to it and feel as if I already had it. I didn't know how it was going to work at the time, but in my heart, I believed it would. My dream was to be working with Reiki, to share the energies and my passion for it and eventually teach it to others so that it could help them too, if they were needing help. The manifesting worked and my dream was about to come true.

Two years after starting this job, the workplace was closing down permanently and I knew this was the perfect opportunity to finally start my own business and work with Reiki.

For anyone wishing to learn how to manifest their dreams, desires or wishes, I do recommend reading the book and working with its techniques. For me, the more I noticed the changes coming into my life through manifestation, the more confident I became in using it. And the more I began using it, the more I believed in its power. The more I believed in its power, the more I began to manifest. Now, it has just become part of me. I use these techniques naturally all the time,. And now, instead of wondering if it's going to happen, I get excited about when its going to happen and then I let go of becoming too attached to the outcome and just trust in the process.

Here's a more detailed look at how this works for me:

MANIFESTING DIARY

The very first step that I took after reading the book was to get a large notebook as my Manifesting Diary. Every night before bed, I list all the things I am grateful for on one page. This tends to reflect what has happened during the day, as well as my gratitude for family, and friends and my surroundings. On the opposite page, I list all the things, that I wish to manifest. Instead of writing it as something I wish for I write in the present tense as if I already have it and I am grateful for it. So I start each sentence with "Thank you for …." or "I am am truly grateful to have ……in my life".

I write long lists every night filling, each page of the diary. The page of gratitude, with the things that I am manifesting tends to repeat, but I do it every night, adding more strength and power to what I was wanting. Some of these things are very small and some are very large. Whenever I look through my Manifesting Diary, I smile and give thanks as I have received it all that I have received all that I have wished for over the years.

VISUALISATION

The next step for me is visualisation. I did struggle a bit with this one at first, but I persevered and over time it got easier. There are different ways that I do this. One is to visualise actually having what I was manifesting whilst writing my gratitude for it in the diary. Another way, is by taking some time out and sitting still, imagining it in my mind's eye. What I have found as time has gone on is that the manifestation process happens quicker when I still my mind and visualise what I want while feeling as if I already have it and sensing how I feel now that it is mine.

Another way - especially good for those for whom mental visualisation is difficult or impossible - is with pictures, in the past I have made picture collages and hung them in a place I could see them often. Nowadays, when there I something I want to manifest, I put a picture on the screen saver that's on my phone. This means I am consciously and subconsciously seeing it every time I pick up my phone. It's all about finding a way that works for you. My daughter makes visualisation boards, and these work great for her. She cuts out pictures of what she wants and puts it on her board, leaving her board on the wall in a prominent place where she can see it. This works very well for her; she always gets everything that is on her vision board. When she has all these things, she changes her pictures to make and manifest her new wish list.

FAITH AND CLARITY

What I have found over the years is the more that I have manifested - and believe me it's a lot, including a whole new me - the easier it has become. Once you start to see the results, your belief system becomes stronger and something within your heart just knows that you're going to receive what you want. You begin creating your own reality. Maybe you don't always get it as you expect, but you do receive it.

A bit of advice I would give when doing this is to be careful about what it is you are asking for. Here is an example of receiving what I wanted but not how I wanted it. I once I asked for more flowers in my life. I wasn't specific I just asked for more flowers in my life. What happened next was that someone left a flower on my car windscreen - every day for six weeks. The first day it happened, I was delighted. But as time went on it actually began to frighten me, so much so I would try to stay awake all night just to find out who was doing it. Eventually I did find out, and it was a rather creepy experience. It did stop, but not before leaving me with a lot of stress. Please don't let this story stop you being creative with manifesting though, everything is an experience to be learnt from.

INTENTION

These steps provide a great way to begin, they reflect how I began my manifesting experiences. Since then I have found various different ways to manifest - and I'm sure you will too. Later on in life, when I had my Holistic Centre, everyone that worked there would meet up on a full moon. We would get together, and each of us would write a list, things that we were holding on to and wanting to let go of and a list of all the things we wanted to bring into our life. Then we would do a group meditation that included letting go of what no longer served us and, bringing forth our wishes and desires. We had a lot of fun doing this and I think the power of many people doing it together makes the energies stronger. Everything is about intention, and during my Reiki classes I also show people how to manifest what they wish for with Reiki.

Nowadays, I truly believe that saying your intention out aloud to someone is the first step in bringing it forth. I have great faith in the ability of manifestation to work by setting intentions and absolutely believing that you already have it.

Using the methods, I began to manifest everything I desired. I changed myself and my life, creating my life, rather than just living it and allowing it to create me. I choose my reality and I can now understand how certain things in my past happened, as I did not have that control over my life, at that time.

My advice to anyone wanting to start this process would be: think of it as the law of attraction - what you think becomes your reality, so be very aware of your thoughts and what it is you're imagining. Thoughts become things. Be careful about what you wish for and always speak in the positive - being aware of what you are saying is important. Intention is an important step to. Focusing your intention towards something you wish to create and knowing what you want makes all the difference. Once you know, say it out loud, write it, visualise it, have gratitude for it, Reiki it, have positive intention for it, meditate on it, feel it, allow yourself feelings of joy around it and put love to it, like you already have it. You can play about with this and do what feels right for you, but definitely put your intention and attention to it. Everything is energetic, so be aware of your frequency, raise your vibration.

Don't try and work out how your manifestation will happen, just allow it to happen. Some things can be instant, some take days or weeks, months or even years - just trust and believe it will happen and it will. It is good to show gratitude when you do receive it and also to have a note of everything that you achieve through positive intention and manifestation. This allows your belief to grow and your confidence in achieving it will also grow.

Happy manifesting. !!!

The next chapter goes into a manifestation, that I wished for and wrote in my diary every night for nearly two years: to have my own business and work with the Reiki energies.

AWAKENING THE INNER LIGHT

AFFIRMATIONS/MANTRAS

- I welcome signs and synchronicities as guidance on my path.
- My soul is always expanding into its fullest expression.
- I trust the timing of my spiritual awakening.
- I am both the student and the teacher of my own journey.
- The universe supports my growth in every moment.

EMPOWERING HEALING SUGGESTIONS/TECHNIQUES

1. SYNCHRONICITY JOURNAL - Record repeating numbers, symbols, dreams, or signs you notice, and reflect other meaning.
2. MANIFESTATION MORNING - Start each day by visualising one thing you wish to call in, as if it's already here.
3. CLARITY CANDLE RITUAL - Light a white candle and focus on your intention, allowing the flame to "burn away" doubt.
4. ENERGY EXPANSION PRACTISE - Sit in meditation and imagine your energy field growing brighter and larger with each breath.
5. FAITH IN ACTION - Take one small inspired step each week toward your dreams, even if you don't know the outcome.

JOURNALING REFLECTION QUESTIONS

- How do I recognise spiritual growth in my life?

- What signs or synchronicities have felt especially meaningful to me?

- How do I currently manifest my desires?

- What new spiritual practises feel exciting to explore?

- Where in my life could I lean more into faith and trust?

- Additional reflection or memories that surface.

BECOMING

You are not who you once were.
You are a river, finding new bends.
A sky, opening to wider horizons.

At first, the change is quiet -
A feather landing on water,
A seed turning in the dark.
But inside the roots begin to drink,
And the branches reach higher.

Signs arrive like whispered invitations -
A feather in your path,
A song at the perfect time,
A dream you can't forget.
The universe is speaking in a language
Your soul has always known.

You are the seeker
And the one who is found.
You are both questioning answer,
Shadow and light,

Each step you take
Is a prayer,
Each breath yes, to becoming.

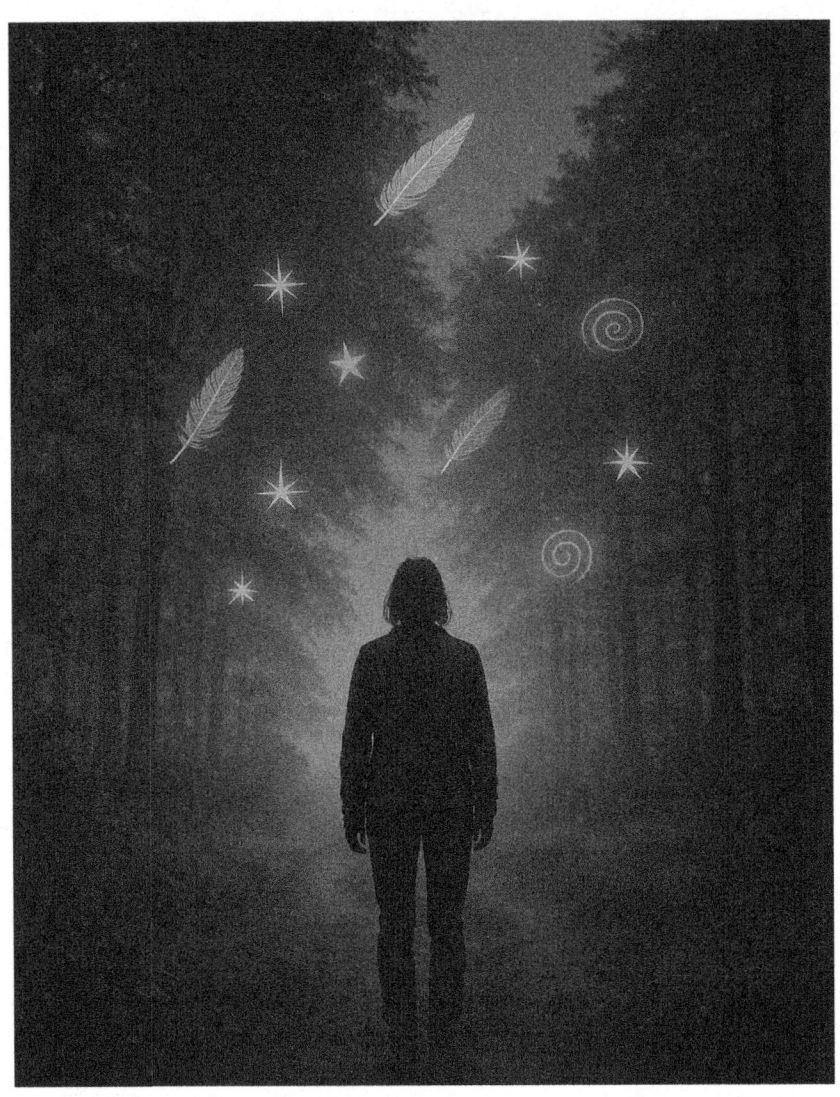

Awakening the Inner Light

CHAPTER 4 - THE BIRTH OF TRANQUILITY

A couple of months before turning 40 - and 12 years after becoming unwell - my life had changed completely and I became self-employed, running my own business and working with Reiki as well as other therapies that I had trained in. This made me so happy.

My health was so much better, but I still tended to dip into days when I felt unwell again. Sometimes this lasted a couple of days, sometimes much longer. I had to be careful, with and make sure not to overdo things. I still had a lot to learn and as the years went on I was sent many more lessons about things that I had to change and overcome. Having my dream business helped with this, and I could also work the hours that suited me - and work around my family's needs.

After my last workplace closed down and I realised I would be out of work, I spoke with my husband about having my own business and working from home. He understood how unhappy I had been in my last job and realised how passionate I was about helping people with Reiki and massage. So we agreed to look into having a log cabin in the back garden. This would mean people could come and go through the garden without disrupting our home life or any of our neighbours. I did a lot of research to find out how to run a business from home and what I could and couldn't have in the garden. When I completed the research and contacted all the different parties required, we got a loan and built the log cabin. I knew exactly how I wanted it to look as I had spent a lot of time visualising it. When I described it my husband, he was able to build it to my specifications. It was a lot of hard work at the time, and I was lucky that he was very good at this type of work. The garden was unrecognisable at one point as we had wood lying everywhere and had to dig a six-foot trench for wastepipes to the cabin.

The finished result was amazing. The log cabin had a toilet, sinks, shelving, a waiting room and a treatment room. The feel inside was wonderful; the smell and energy of the wood made it very special and you could feel this as soon as you entered. I got it all kitted out with matching colours and had salt lamps and dimmed lighting to create the right ambience.

Now that the log cabin was ready, I had to name my business and start advertising for clients. After a lot of deliberation, I decided to name the business "Tranquility". I designed leaflets showing my services and had an open day to show people around and let them know what was on offer. The open day was a success and lots of people showed up. Many became my first clients.

At the beginning of my new venture, I was nervous every time someone booked in for a treatment, but as soon as I started working I felt totally in my comfort zone and really enjoyed it. It took years to build up my business but as time went on, it did grow and so did I. Everything about me was changing and I was constantly learning new skills. I thanked the universe for every person that walked through those doors.

As the years went on my health began to improve. I even began exercising again and I was certainly changing my lifestyle. I was changing mentally, emotionally, physically and spiritually. Even when I wasn't working I would be down in the log cabin doing work on my spiritual self. I would go down there to meditate, journal, read and study. The calming atmosphere of the log cabin really made a difference to me.

In 2013, I decided I was ready to train as a Reiki teacher. I wished to be able to spread the gift of Reiki to others and to share everything that I had learnt over the years. I never had enough money to be able to do the Reiki Master and Reiki Teachers course's, but every night I would write in my Manifesting Diary. "Thank you for being a Reiki teacher". On 23rd December 2013, my dream was about to come true.

At this time, my son played rugby for the local rugby team, which had a monthly lottery draw; you paid a fee for your number and if it came up you won £400. That particular day, we were getting ready to go as a family to George Square in Glasgow to see the Christmas lights. We did this every year just before Christmas to soak up the atmosphere. It was something we all enjoyed and watching the children get excited for Christmas Day was such a pleasure. Just as we were leaving to go to Glasgow, the house telephone rang and I answered it; it was the Helensburgh Rugby Club to say that I had won the lottery. But that was not all - it had been a three-month rollover and there was a cheque for £1,200 waiting on me. I can't even put into words how I felt, I danced around the living room; I sang (badly I may add, as anyone who knows me will testify); I laughed; and I cried. The joy and gratitude I felt was immense; I could now do my Reiki Masters and `Reiki Teachers course.

On 2nd February, 2014, I completed my Master's course then worked towards my Teacher's course. iI was a lot of work and I had to write four Reiki manuals, one for each level, but I enjoyed it very much. I poured all my love and knowledge into those manuals, and on 25th March, 2014, I qualified was a Reiki Teacher, 10 years after learning Reiki One.

I began letting people know that I was now teaching Reiki and I did get from in others learning it. At that time, I would only do one-on-one teaching or occasionally two people at the same time. I still suffered from shyness then, but, I now teach larger classes. I love each class as much as I loved doing the very first class. I feel totally in my comfort zone running a Reiki class. I have heard so many stories over the years about how it changes people's lives; it truly is amazing. One thing I have noticed is that each class always has the right amount of people in it and always has the right people for each class. They normally have something in common with each other, so that the people in that class end up bonding so well.

The more I worked with Reiki, the more my intuition grew. This lead me to start reading Tarot cards and I began offering readings as part of my services. I did training on meditation and mindfulness and began running meditation classes at Tranquility. I would take a maximum of four people at that time for these classes. I was getting further and further into my spiritual work, learning and teaching as I went along. My health was improving, but I was getting terrible issues with my abdomen and a lot of pain.

I went to the doctor about these problems and after a while went for a colonoscopy. The procedure involves putting a camera up your rectum and into the colon so the doctor can see if there is anything going on. This ended up being quite a traumatic experience for me. The day I went for the colonoscopy, I felt dehydrated, as I wasn't allowed to eat or drink from the night before. When I got to my appointment, I was taken to the treatment room and had a needle put into my arm to give me a sedative for the procedure. Every time they tried to put the needle into my arm, my veins would collapse. They tried various different veins, and several different medical personnel had a go, but with no luck. After a lengthy time of this going on, I was given the option of getting it done without the sedative or coming back another day to try again. I decided to get it over and done with without the sedative - a decision I came to regret and certainly would not recommend to anyone. The pain I felt was awful. I watched the screen that showed you what the camera was seeing and, I even watched as they cut a couple of polyps off to get tested. I was so glad when it was all over. I ended up in bed very unwell for a couple of weeks after this. The M.E. symptoms hit me with a vengeance.

I can't remember now how long it took to get my results, but I do remember being disappointed by them. I was told that I either had irritable bowel syndrome (IBS) or it was endometriosis which I had been diagnosed with a few years previously, that was causing the pain. I was told I could get further investigations if I went to the gynaecologist again. I made the decision that I wasn't going to do this as the endometriosis diagnosis had involved a minor operation under general anaesthetic and I didn't want to go through that again.

After leaving the hospital, I decided that I was going to find out as much as I could about nutrition and see if I could heal my body this way. This was another big lesson that I was about to learn.

I threw myself into learning about nutrition and began eliminating a lot of foods from my diet. Instead of taking this slowly and changing one thing at a time, I was all in. This did have an effect on my body at first, as I was making too many changes at the one time, but after a lengthy process, and a lot of experimenting, I found what agreed with my body. I cut out sugar, gluten, diary, meat and fish. This works well for me, and I have stayed with this process to this day. I can have the occasional bit of food that has sugar or gluten but I try not to deviate from my eating plan as it really agrees with my body. I also drink lots of water.

Making the changes was difficult at first as I craved the types of food I used to eat, but as time went on I found I craved the healthier options and now I'm at a stage where I couldn't go back to the way I used to eat. The changes that happened when I made the modifications to my diet were amazing. I had no more pain or bloating. My energy levels soared, and I felt so much better about myself. I was able to increase the amount of physical exercise that I did and I even joined a gym and began to get fit again.

Changing my diet was a big piece of the jigsaw puzzle and made a huge difference to my health. A day that I will never ever forget in my life was 1st October, 2017, I ran a 10k in the Glasgow Great North Run. Not only did I complete it, but I got a time of just under one hour. The atmosphere was electric, and I could hear the crowds of people clapping and cheering everyone on. As I neared the finish line, I was struggling and praying that I wouldn't collapse over it. My legs felt like jelly and I was concentrating on just putting one foot in front of the other. The feeling of joy and bliss that came over me when I finally crossed the finishing line, meant everything to me; even now as I write this I feel tears of joy and happiness welling up in my eyes. I will never, ever forget that feeling. After the race, I went home and lay in the bath and cried and cried; these were happy tears. I had won; going from lying in bed, barely able to walk some days to running a 10k, 19 years later. It had been a long battle to recover from this illness, but I did it. I was so grateful.

Since this date, I have run a 10k again. I have also done Tough Mudder, which is an endurance event in which participants attempt a 10-12 mile obstacle course. The obstacles include fire, water, electricity and heights. It is a team event and I did it with the gym I belonged to. Today I am still physically active and make the most of this. I think the experience of having this taken away from you makes you so grateful when you are able to be physical again. On days I don't feel like doing physical activity, I think of this and it motivates me to do something. I also think of the good feeling I get after exercising and find that this helps.

Changing my diet made such a difference to me; I would encourage anyone to be aware of what they are feeding their body. Having now learnt about nutrition, I know it is important to get the balance and find out what agrees with your body. What you put into your body, makes a difference to how well your body works. I would highly recommend anyone who is unwell or wanting more energy to have a look at their diet and make changes. Having a healthy gut is so important. What I would say is don't try and do everything at once, but make small changes and watch the difference it makes - even keep a diary of how you feel after eating certain food groups and see what works well for you. Also be prepared; write a shopping list before you go shopping and stick to it; have a menu plan for the week and stick to it; cook from scratch whenever you can.

Advice that I would give to anyone wanting to transition to a healthier diet:

- Drink lots of water. Replace any sugary drinks with water and watch your alcohol intake; alcohol dehydrates the body and has a high sugar content.

- Increase your intake of fruit and vegetables. You can do this is by snacking on fruit if you're feeling hungry, filling your plate with lots of vegetables or salad and making soup with lots of vegetables. Make sure when you increase your fruit and vegetables that you choose a wide variety. Experiment with them. The more you eat them, the more you begin to crave them.

- Cut sugar and processed foods from your diet. Learn to make things from scratch and find healthier alternatives. As well as snacking on fruits, nuts and seeds are good options.

- Don't buy diet foods; a lot of them have more additives in them and you need healthy fats for your body. Have a look at the labels of different foods. Being aware of what you're putting in your body, will make such a difference.

- Eat more whole grains. You can swap white rice for brown rice, white bread for a wholegrain bread.

- Use healthy oils. There are various types. I tend to use coconut and olive oil.

- Increase your protein. You can do this by adding pulses; use lentils and beans in your cooking.

- Use more fresh herbs in your cooking. Different herbs have different benefits and are also a flavoursome way to change the taste of your meals.

- Most importantly, find out what works for your body. Everybody is different, so take it slowly and find out what helps make your body work more efficiently.

My tips for boosting your energy are: drink more water, change your diet, get more quality sleep, limit alcohol, avoid smoking, avoid stress as much as possible, don't take on more than your body can handle, and move more.

Something that I have noticed is that one of the best things you can do for your body is to get outdoors. Walking is wonderful for us and can change how we are feeling. It definitely uplifts us and helps us to feel better; there are so many benefits to walking outdoors.

Be the best version of you!!

Over a matter of months in 2017, several clients asked me why I was "hiding in the back garden". I took this as a sign and decided to make another life-changing decision; I would open a Holistic Centre in town.

STEPPING INTO THE DREAM

AFFIRMATIONS/MANTRAS

- I am worthy of living my dreams now.
- Courage grows every time I step beyond my comfort zone.
- My healing space radiates love and peace to all who enter.
- I am supported in creating a life I love.
- Fear is just an invitation to grow.

EMPOWERING HEALING SUGGESTIONS/TECHNIQUES

1. COMFORT ZONE CHALLENGE - Once a week, do one small thing that stretches you beyond what feels familiar.
2. VISION BOARD FOCUS - Create a visual representation of your dream life and place it somewhere you will see daily.
3. SACRED SPACE BLESSING - Smudge your home or workspace with sage, palo Santo, or incense while speaking loving intentions.
4. NUTRITION UPGRADE - Add one healing nutrient-rich food to your meals each day and notice the difference.
5. DAILY FEAR CHECK-IN - Write down one fear that's coming uo and reframe it into an empowering belief.

JOURNALING REFELCTION QUESTIONS

- What fears have kept me from pursuing my dreams?

- How does it feel to imagine myself already living that dream?

- What practical steps could I take to bring my vision closer?

- How does my environment support or hinder my healing?

- What part of my comfort zone am I ready to release?

- Additional reflection or memories that surface.

THE THRESHOLD

There comes a moment
When the door you've been staring at
For months, years, a lifetime -
Begins to open.

It creaks with the weight
Of all the times you almost stepped through
But didn't.
It smells of fresh beginnings
And faint traces of your own courage.

On the other side
Is not just a dream, but a homecoming.
A place you have been building
In the quiet of the corners of your heart.

Yes fear lingers at the edge.
Yes, your hands tremble.
Bt your soul is steady. It knows the path.
It planted this seed long before you knew its name.

Step forward.
Feel the light catch your face.
This is the moment
You stop waiting and start living.

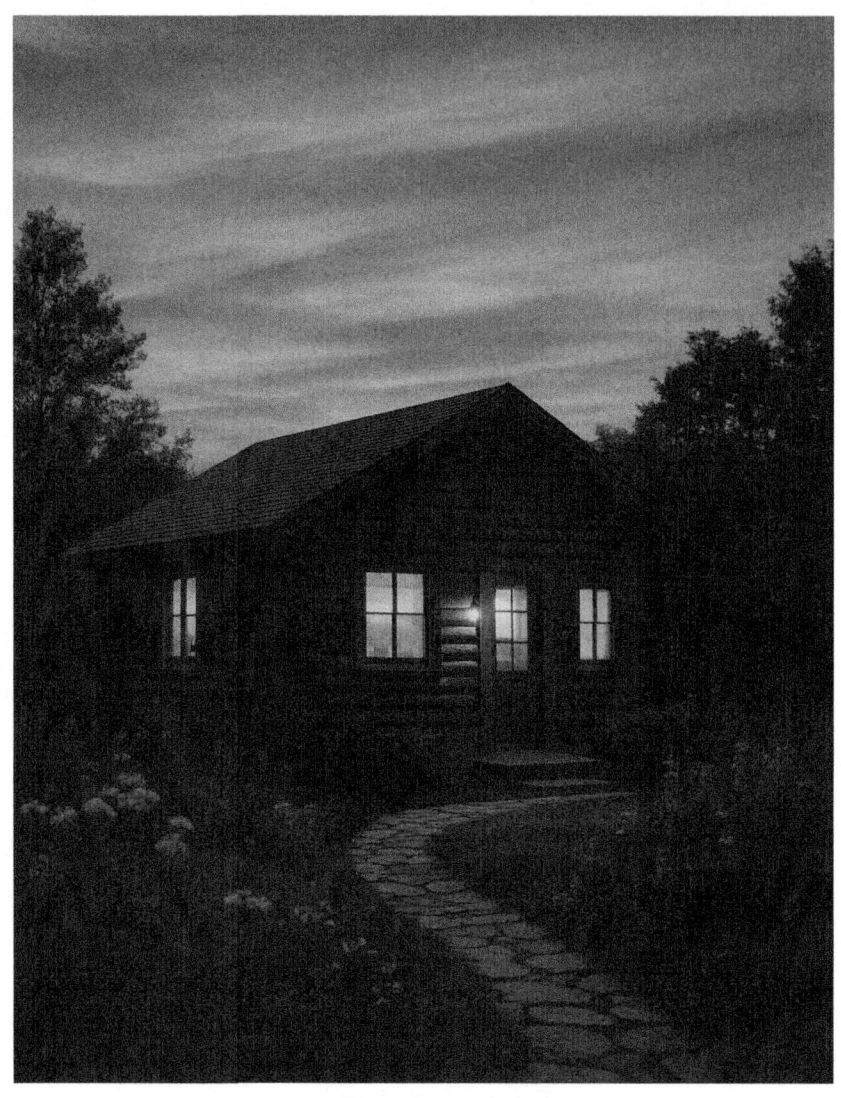

Stepping into the Dream

CHAPTER 5 - TRANQUILITY HOLISTIC CENTRE

I loved Tranquility; I loved the setting, I enjoyed my work, and it was so fulfilling to provide therapies and see the difference it made to others. My health was improving with every passing year and I do think that putting into practise all that I was learning made all the difference. I listened to my body and what it needed, but I was also listening to my soul and doing my very best to follow my heart. I paid attention to signs that were all around me and always tried to make sense of them; over the years I have called this talking to the universe, talking to my angels, talking to God, talking to the Reiki energies, talking to Source, following signs, listening to my gut, and tuning into my higher being. I believe you can call it what you wish - but being in touch with that inner self, tuning into yourself, knowing yourself and following what your heart says, makes all the difference. It helps you learn about yourself. I was doing this more and more, and by doing this I was pushing myself, mentally, physically, emotionally and spiritually. I was facing my fears and growing in self-confidence, but to be honest, sometimes the fear actually made me physically sick, although the sense of achievement and growth was worth it.

By the end of 2017, I made a decision that was going to push me completely out of my comfort zone again, but I can honestly say that this was another life-changing decision that would help me to grow even stronger in all ways. I decided to move from Tranquility in the log cabin and open a shop, calling it Tranquility Holistic Centre. I listened to the signs; everything was pushing me in that direction. I was excited, I was scared. In fact, I think I went through every emotion there could possibly be, but I knew I was going to do it. I knew it would be hard work, but I was ready for this.

I began looking for properties to rent early in the new year. I had this sense of urgency; I wanted to open the Holistic Centre right now. As always, my impatience was something that I would have to let go of. I have learned now to be patient (well, far more patient than I ever was) and I do believe everything happens at the right time, so I am better at letting things unfold in their own time. Back then though, I still wanted things right away! The right place did come up at the right time, but I would have to wait until May for this to happen.

Preparing to open a bigger business, was a lot of hard work. I had a vision though, and I spent hours on end working everything out and organising it. I had to prepare a business plan. I had to research data and statistics. I had too work out pricing, open a different business bank account, learn more about advertising, create leaflets and flyers. I had to choose decor and colour schemes and find out what furniture and soft furnishings I would need. I wanted to employ staff to manage my reception, so I had to learn how to do wages, and how to be an employer. I also wanted to let out rooms to other therapists so that the centre could offer a wider variety of therapies. I also wanted a shop within it, with different holistic products for sale. I was quite specific in what I wanted the Holistic Centre to be like. It was a lot of work preparing for it, but I thrived on it. I love learning new things and this was a new, and massive challenge for me. I was determined that it would all work out. I just knew in my heart that this was the right thing to do.

I went to view a couple of different properties that were available for rent, but neither felt right. I was sure that I would know as soon as I walked in to the right place it. I knew if I listened to my heart it would guide me in the right direction.

This is exactly what happened. In May, I went to view a property that had come up for rent and I instantly knew this was it. It had four rooms, a small kitchen, a toilet/washroom and a larger area that could accommodate a reception area with a shop. I agreed to the lease terms, signed the paperwork and then began to get organised for the opening of Tranquility Holistic Centre.

The next few weeks were a whirlwind of craziness. I wanted one of the rooms extended so that workshops and classes could be held in there, and that left three rooms for treatments. Over the next few weeks, I was decorating, organising all the furniture and soft furnishings, finding others to rent the rooms, finding reception staff, advertising and setting up everything else to do with getting the business up and running. On top of this, I was still working, and still training for the Tough Mudder, which I completed in June. And just before the opening, I was going to London for a few days with my son and my mum. Looking back, I don't know how I managed to do it all, but I did, and the best thing was I had the energy to be able to do it.

My opening day was on Saturday, 7th July, 2018. Everyone that would be working there set up their stalls, for the grand opening. We put out refreshments and food, and at 10 a.m. I officially opened the doors to Tranquility Holistic Centre. I did get a bad case of nervousness before this, and was actually sick, but I put on a new beautiful bright orange dress with matching shoes and spent time doing my hair and makeup. For some reason, making the extra effort with my appearance did make me feel more confident. When we were all set and the front door was opened, something came over me - a confidence I had never felt before. I still remember clearly this feeling, and the day was extremely successful. There were bookings in everyone's diaries and there had been a lot of products sold from the shop. The opening day flew by and I was so happy with how everything had gone; it had been a success.

This was the start of my new business, and I loved it. The atmosphere in that place was amazing. I have lots and lots of great memories and experiences from there and it changed me in a way that I will be eternally grateful for. Everything was a learning curve, and I grew and grew in self-confidence, self-belief and self-love, I was definitely changing. It was a busy place, and I worked long hours. Some days I was exhausted by day-end, but I was also grateful that I could work again.

Not only was I providing therapies, I was now running classes. I held Reiki classes, Angelic Reiki classes and Meditation classes, but it wasn't with just one or two people as it had been in the log cabin. I normally had about six people in each class. At first I was nervous about running the classes, but as time went on my nerves began to lessen. Because I was so passionate about what I was teaching, it didn't feel like work. I loved what I was teaching and I loved watching the difference it made to people's lives.

We were like a family in there, and each full moon, everyone that worked there would get together. We would sit in a circle in the larger room and have an altar with candles placed on it. Everyone brought their own crystals and we would place them on the altar on top of our manifestation lists, on one side of the paper we would write what we would like to let go of and on the other side we would write what we wished to bring into our lives. I would lead a full moon meditation and then we would then choose angel cards from different packs that people brought in and read their meanings out aloud. These cards always had relevant advice and seemed to say what that particular person was needing to hear at that particular time. Sometimes we would also do some drumming. These nights were magical, and I think that we all needed them. They helped each of us in different ways, but ways that we needed.

As well as teaching meditation, I practised it all the time. I feel meditation is another useful tool that everyone should use for self-development. Taking the time to quieten the mind is so important and has so many benefits. When you make meditation part of your daily practise it can bring about several changes in your emotional and physical being.

Here are some of the benefits of meditation I have noticed in myself and others:

- it can help you to focus on the present moment. When you focus on the present moment, you let go of thoughts of the past (which can contribute to depression) and you let go of thoughts of the future (which helps you let go of anxiety).

- It helps you to gain a new perspective on stressful situations. When your head is full of thoughts going round and round, sometimes your judgement or problem-solving becomes clouded. When you quieten the mind, it allows help and solutions to come to the forefront.

- It can reduce negative emotions and allow you an increased sense of self-awareness.

- It can help increase your imagination and creativity because you aren't scattering your thoughts everywhere; you are practising bringing focused intention.

- It gives you the skills to manage your stress levels and along with that increases your patience and tolerance.

- It can lower your resting heart rate and your blood pressure. Your sleep quality may also improve.

Research into meditation suggests that it can help with lots of different medical complaints, including, anxiety, depression, chronic pain, asthma, cancer, heart disease, high blood pressure, irritable bowel syndrome, tension headaches and sleep problems.

There are various different types of meditation including, mindfulness meditation, spiritual meditation, mantra meditation, movement meditation, focused meditation, transcendental meditation, guided meditation and loving kindness meditation.

If you are new to meditation, I would suggest taking it slowly. Don't be hard on yourself; it can take a long time to master meditation. Your brain is a muscle and like any other muscle in your body it takes time to train a muscle; repetition is key. Experiment with different types of meditation and see what works best for you. Set yourself a certain amount of time each day to bring this into practise. You can start with as little as a minute a day and add to this time as the days go on. Setting the intention to make time for you every day is beneficial in making meditation a habit.

I also believe meditating, in the same place everyday is good. You may have a favourite chair, that you can use that. If it feels right for you, light candles, place crystals around you, or do anything that makes this feel like your special "me time". It is worth the effort and will be so beneficial to you.

Meditation is an important element in self-care and with practise you will get better at it and see the benefits.

Tranquility Holistic Centre taught me so much and definitely changed me as a person but things were to change, yet again, when we went into lockdown in 2020.

EXPANDING INTO POSSIBILITY

AFFIRMATIONS/MANTRAS

- I am capable of leading with both strength and compassion.
- My work uplifts and inspires everyone it touches.
- I am confident in my ability to grow and succeed.
- I attract the right people, opportunities, and blessings.
- Every challenge is an invitation to expand my light.

EMPOWERING HEALING SUGGESTIONS/TECHNIQUES

1. CONFIDENCE ANCHOR - Before important conversations or events, place your hand over your solar plexus and affirm, "I'm powerful and capable."
2. TEAM ENERGY CLEARING - If working with others, open each meeting with a short grounding or gratitude practise.
3. SACRED WORKSPACE RESET - Regularly declutter and energetically cleanse your work environment.
4. GROWTH MINDSET PRACTISE - Replace "I can't" with "I'm learning to ….."
5. COMMUNITY BLESSING RITUAL - Light a candle each week and set intentions for those you serve, sending out ripples of positive energy.

JOURNALING REFLECTION QUESTIONS

- How has stepping into my role in work changed me?

- What strengths have I discovered through working?

- How can I nurture my confidence while staying grounded ?

- What qualities do I value in those I work with?

- How can my work be both financially sustainable and spiritually fulfilling?

- Additional reflection or memories that surface.

THE GARDEN YOU PLANTED

You began with a single seed -
An idea, dream whispered
On a quiet afternoon.

You watered it with courage
And fed it with faith.
Through storms and sunshine,
You kept tending.

And then one morning
You woke to find a garden-
Doors opening, voices laughing,
Hearts gathering in a shared light.

You became not just the keeper
Of your own gardens, but the guardian
Of a sacred space, where others could grow too.

Every challenge was a stone in the path,
But you built with them -
Stronger walls, wider foundations,
A home for healing.

And now, you stand in the centre of it all,
Knowing that you are the roots and the blossom,
The gardener and the garden.

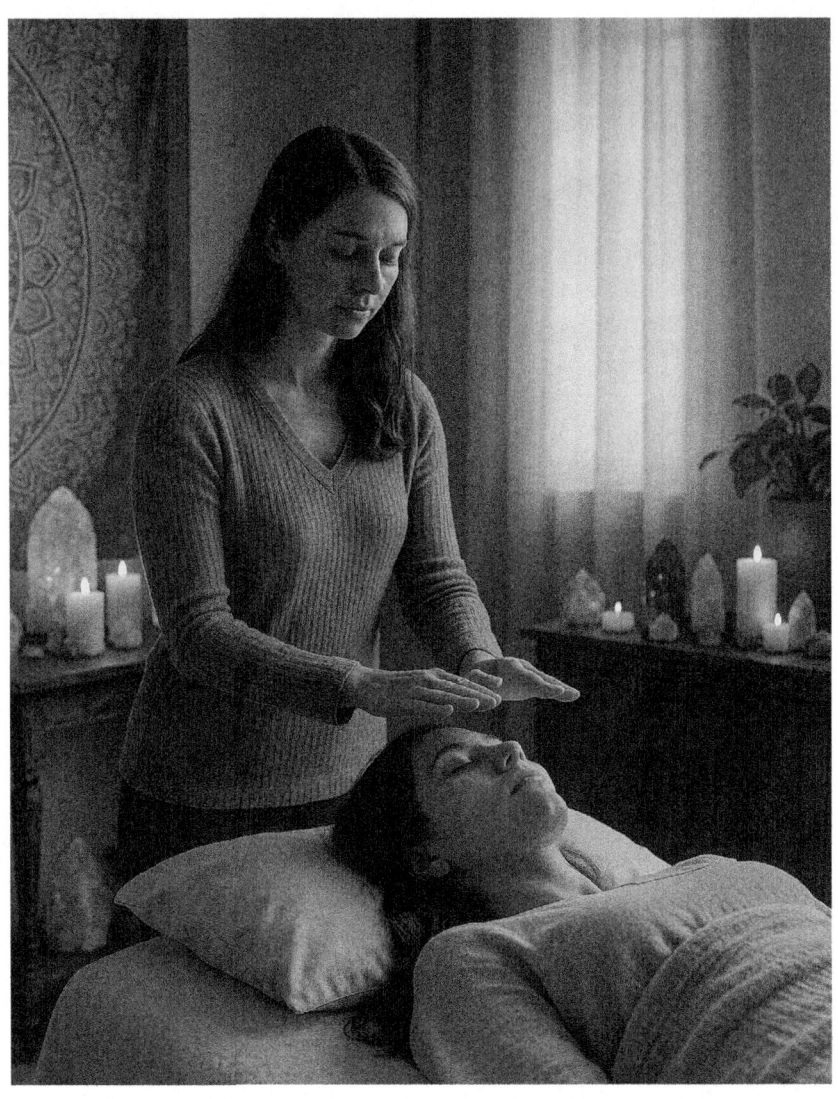
Expanding Into Possibility

CHAPTER 6 - THE DIVORCE

In October 2019, my husband and I separated. We were still living together until a separation agreement was agreed. This was a very difficult period, but at least I had Tranquility Holistic Centre. It was my saviour as I threw myself into my work, working more and more hours. We came to a separation agreement at the turn of 2020, just as a lot of people began taking unwell with Covid and a lot of people stopped going to public places in fear of catching it.

Under the terms of the separation agreement, my husband was going to continue to live in our house and I was moving out. It wasn't really what I had wanted but I didn't want to fight about the separation and I needed things to be as easy as possible as the stress was making me unwell again. I found a flat and the entry date was 4th April, 2020. I was struggling to keep going and all the symptoms of M.E. were flaring up again. I just wanted to make my life easier. Then it all changed in March 2020, when we saw the whole world go into lockdown.

On 21st March my life was turned upside down. I had to close my business as the country went into lockdown. The weeks leading up to this had been extremely difficult, as fewer and fewer clients came in, but this was the day everything came crashing down on me. I learned I had no business and no money. I was unable to move on the 4th April, and so I was stuck in my house in lockdown with my ex-husband. My daughter had had her second son in January and I couldn't see or help her with my grandsons. My son was still at home and had to live in this terrible atmosphere that had grown between my ex-husband and me. This period of my life was extremely difficult.

My body couldn't cope with all the stress, and I became so ill that I was in bed for three weeks. As I lay there, exhausted, I began putting everything that I had learned into practise, but now on a bigger scale. I had time to reflect and time to begin healing myself. There was no way I could go back to my life the way it was all those years ago when I was at the height of my illness.

Everyday, I did Reiki, mediated, wrote in my Manifesting Diary, prayed, wrote positive affirmations and journaled. I worked hard on myself and did everything I could to get into a positive mindset; deep in my heart I knew everything would work out. I believe that everything happens for a reason, although some days this felt hard to accept. I kept working on myself and I did get better and things did change. In May I got money that was owed to me. This meant I could use this money to move, pay the bills and have food on my table.

On 22nd May 2020, I got the keys to my new flat. We were still in lockdown, but I was able to move. I took the few belongings I had and started my new life in the flat. At first it was as if I had a new lease of life. I would put on some music and dance, but as the time went on I began to feel lonely.

From the age of 21, I had been a full-time mum and now I had all this time and didn't know what to do with myself. It's very difficult when you've kept extremely busy with family life and looking after everyone else for 29 years and then, in what seems like a blink of an eye, your family have all grown up and are doing their own thing. It's even more challenging when you have split with someone you have lived with and loved for over quarter of a century and you now find yourself away from the home that you cherished and cared for over twenty five years - a home where you raised your children - and now it is no longer yours and everything has changed. I was having to start all over again and, to be honest, I was a bit lost.

I didn't realise at this time what a transitional period this was, and its only on reflecting on it now that I see that it was massive; everything had changed practically overnight and my life was nothing like what I had been used to. Everything was different. I do think now that I should've taken some time to grieve over this, but as I always do, I put my head up, put a smile on my face and pretended that everything was alright. I do wonder why we do this to ourselves. Why do we always put on a brave face and let no-one know what we are feeling, including ourselves? I would be the first person to listen and support anyone that opened up to me, but for some reason I have always kept my feelings and worries to myself instead of sharing this with family and friends, who I know would be happy to listen or help.

Four months after lockdown, we were allowed to go back to work but, nothing was the same at Tranquility Holistic Centre. Everyone's life had changed during this period and a lot of people had made changes to their lives. I was now letting out treatment rooms only very occasionally, meaning I no longer had an income from that. It took a long time for a lot of clients to come in again, and financially I was struggling to pay the overheads for the shop and the bills at my flat. I could no longer afford to pay staff. I had to change the way I worked.

As the weeks and months went by, I did begin to get busy again but, it was difficult as I had no help anymore and was doing everything all by myself. As the year went on, I found myself exhausted again. Then on 26th December 2020 we went into another lockdown. At first, I found it difficult having so much time on my own. Then I came to a decision; I would embrace this as a time for me to reflect, do lots of internal work and make some changes, mind, body and soul. I did a lot of journalling, digging deep into my thoughts and feelings and doing the inner work on myself.

I also signed up with a local coach for a health and fitness programme, all done online and via telephone calls. I kept a diary of everything I ate, following the coach's advice about daily calorie intake. I walked a minimum of 10,000 steps every day. (Some days this proved difficult, with the typical wet and windy Scottish winter, but I just put on the appropriate clothing, listened to music on my earphones and walked and walked). I had an exercise programme to follow, which I did at home and I kept a diary of my weight and measurements to record my progress, which I shared with my coach in our weekly phone call catch-ups. It was a 12-week programme and by the end of it I felt so good about myself. I had lots of energy and enjoyed having the time to follow the exercises and walking each day. Having someone to mentor and encourage me, someone to report to, did make all the difference for me. I also did a couple of courses online at this time; one was for life coaching and the other was for nutrition.

After four months of the second lockdown, it was now April 2021 and time to go back to work - time to start building my business again. And just like after the first lockdown, it was very slow to start I was still doing everything solo. I did decide though that I would love to have a break away. I had never been away on a girls' holiday and in June 2021 I went on my first girlie holiday. This was so exciting, now in my fifties I was going on a girls' trip. Three of us were going and at first we wanted to go overseas, but because of all the restrictions that had been put in place we decided to go to Brighton, in the south of England.

That holiday was amazing. I'm smiling now as I write this. We got the train - well actually three trains, with changes in different cities. We had our packed lunches and beverages all prepared for the journey and we laughed from the minute we got on the first train all the way to Brighton. We arrived at the hotel around 6 p.m. and loved it. The hotel was situated on the front at Brighton overlooking the English Channel, and Brighton Pier was only a five- minute walk away. The sun was shining when we arrived. We put our cases our rooms, and sat outside taking in the stunning view, and raised our cocktail glasses with a great big "Cheers".

We had the most wonderful week. We laughed a lot, ate good food, did lots of sightseeing and danced a lot. Our hotel had a live singer on from late afternoon, and they always sang outside, encouraging everyone to get up and dance. Of course we did just that. Passer'by's would join in too and cars would hoot and beep as they passed by, seeing everyone dancing, singing and having fun. By the time it finished at 9 p.m. we were ready for our beds. Two of us got tattoos while we were there; mine was the business logo, I had used since the day I first opened Tranquility. I have to say I came back from that holiday feeling like a teenager and extremely happy.

Around the same time, I got into a new relationship. This was very daunting at first. Having not dated anyone in nearly 30 years, my head was full of worries and insecurities. I shouldn't have worried because it made me feel good about myself. I hadn't been looking for anyone and had not even considered dating or being in a relationship. It all happened very quickly and we got on really well, having a lot of the same interests and a similar outlook on life. As the year went on, I felt I was working constantly but never having any money left over for myself once the bills for running the business were paid. The punishing work schedule took its toll, and I had went from feeling so good about myself when I had gone back to work in April to now getting all the symptoms of M.E. coming back yet again.

I had a week off work between Christmas and New Year of 2021 and after a lot of reflection, I knew I couldn't possibly continue the way I was going, otherwise I would be right back to square one. This led me to make another life changing decision - this one was massive.

In October of 2021, my new partner had spent six weeks travelling around Europe in a little camper van. This was something I had always wanted to do. He had been in touch with me every day and so I got to see all the places that he was visiting. The decision I made at the end of the year was that I was going to take a year off and go travelling. I thought, if not now, when?

I decided that I would put my flat up for rent, close my business at the end of the financial year, which was the beginning of April, and go travelling. I thought I could work as I was on my travels and set up my business online. I didn't quite work out like that. In January 2022, a friend visited. I'll never forget the date as it was my birthday and we sat having a cup of tea and she said "Why don't you just sell your flat?" This remark put my head in a spin. I got this feeling of absolute fear in my gut as I thought about it. It kept me awake all night and it was all I could think about over the next few days. The fear in my gut was getting stronger, and I knew I had to face this fear; somehow. I knew this was the right thing to do. I considered all the information about renting my flat out to tenants and all the information about selling my flat, and I decided to put my flat up for sale.

This was a difficult decision for me, but I felt it was the right thing to do. It was difficult for me, my family and my friends too, but they did support me as I started the sale process and began closing down my business. Having just built up my possessions, after having to start over again, I began to give everything away again. I was letting my heart drive me. I was tuning into my intuition. I knew this was the right thing to do; it was yet another step on my path to self-growth and as scary as it was, I was doing it.

During this period of busyness I still found the time to meditate and journal. Journaling has been so important to me and I would recommend it to anyone wanting to dig deep and find out more about themselves. Journaling has helped me find the authentic me after giving myself to everyone else over the years. I think that having a family and commitments sees you putting everyone else's needs before your own, so over time you forget what it is that you need and what you like. All of a sudden, you are having to rediscover who you are.

For anyone who wishes to begin journaling, but doesn't know where to start, I would say there is no right or wrong way. As for me, I have a large notepad. Every time I journal, I date the page and simply begin to write. Sometimes I do it after meditating, and I just write what I am feeling. Sometimes I write a question that I want to know the answer to, then I take a deep breath and just start writing whatever comes into my head. Another way that I do it is by picking an angel card, looking at it and writing what I feel it is saying to me. I change the way I do journaling by how I feel on the day, but one thing that always happens is that when I start writing I just write and write without putting thought into it - just allowing the pen to lead the way. It's really interesting to read back what you've written. I have always dated my journal entries so I can look back and see the differences that have occurred.

You have to do what feels right for you. Experiment with it, get your feelings or thoughts down on paper or do some automatic writing; it is very healing and a good way to let go of pent-up emotions or to begin to discover things about yourself.

I would definitely encourage journaling. You'll find out more about you and rediscover yourself!!

At the end of March 2022, I closed my business and by the end of April, I had left Helensburgh to begin my travels.

FINDING MYSELF IN THE QUIET.

AFFIRMATIONS/MANTRAS

- I am whole, even when standing alone.
- Solitude is my sacred space for renewal.
- I release what no longer supports my highest self.
- My own company is a gift I cherish.
- Every ending holds the seed of a new beginning.

EMPOWERING HEALING SUGGESTIONS/TECHNIQUES

1.SACRED SOLITUDE PRACTISE - Spend 15-30 minutes daily without distractions, simply being present with yourself.

2. RELEASING LETTER - Write a letter to what you're letting go of (a person, situation or belief) and burn it safely.

3. HOME SANCTUARY - Choose one corner room to make into a peaceful retreat for meditation, journaling or rest.

4. GRATITUDE LIST - Record one unexpected blessing you discovered during times of stillness.

5. SELF-CARE DATE - Once a week, take yourself somewhere that nurtures you - in a cafe, park, or gallery - just for you.

JOURNALLING REFLECTION QUESTIONS

- What have I learned about myself during time alone?

- What emotions have come up mostly when I am in solitude, and how do I move through them?

- How has my relationship with endings changed?

- What habits or patterns am I ready to release for good?

- What do I now value more deeply about my own company?

- Additional reflection or memories that surface.

THE QUIET THAT HEALS

When the world fell silent,
You heard the voice again -
Soft, unsure at first,
But steady beneath the layers.

The walls around you were not a prison,
But a cocoon. Within them
You learned the shape of your own heart,
The rhythms of your breath,
The places you still needed to tend.

You grieved.
You shed skins.
You met yourself
Without the noise of the worlds demands.

And in the stillness, you found beauty -
A shaft of light through the window,
The way a kettle hums,
The sound of your own laughter returning.

Solitude became your sacred teacher,
Showing you that
You were never truly alone.
The one you had been searching for
Was always here,
Waiting for you to come home.

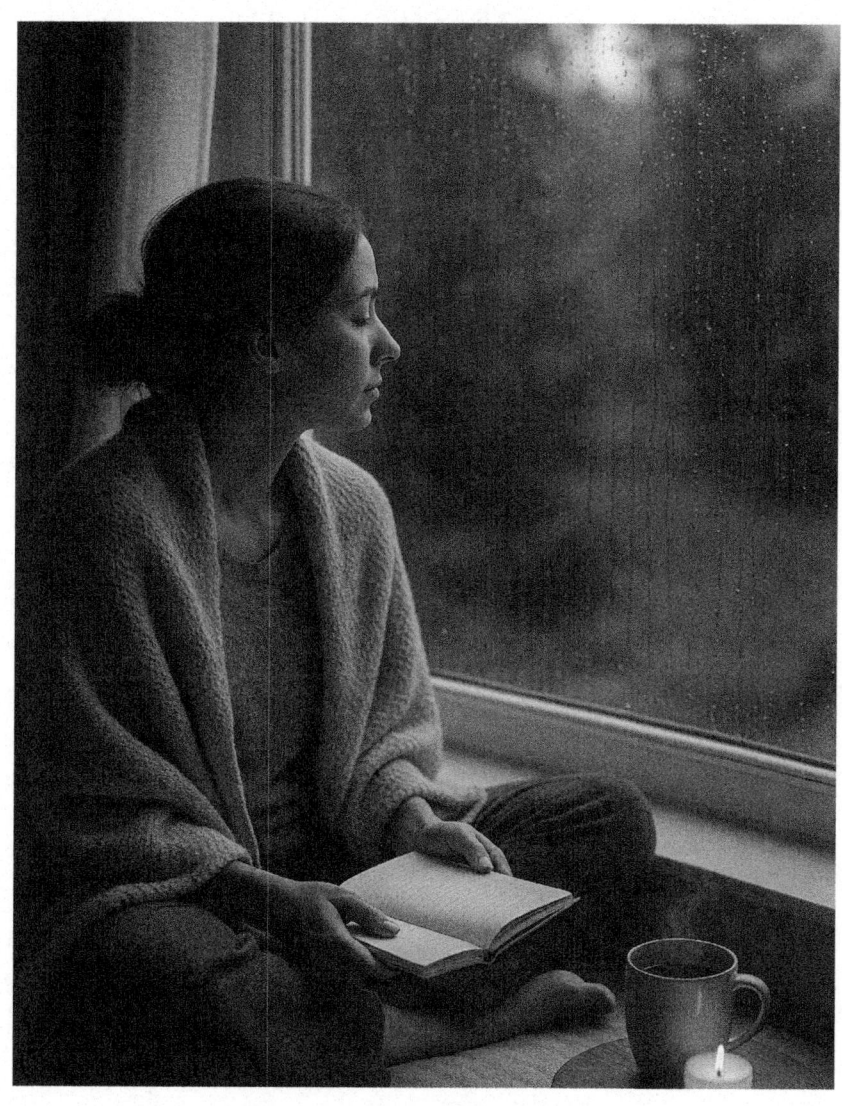
Finding Myself in the Quiet

CHAPTER 7 - THE TRAVELS

Leaving Helensburgh was hard, but at the same time I knew it was temporary and doing it would allow me to go further on my road to self-discovery. There wasn't a plan to follow, only things that I wished to do.

On 28th April, 2022, I handed my keys into the estate agent (my flat had sold quickly), picked up paperwork from the lawyers, filled my car with the few possessions I had, and drove to Berwick-upon-Tweed, North of England, where my partner had a caravan. This caravan was situated in a small caravan park in a field in the middle of nowhere. I wasn't travelling at this on my own at this point; we were doing it together and it felt like a big adventure.

I did like the caravan; the sunrises and sunsets were amazing, I loved the quietness and the relaxing atmosphere, and we were only two miles away from the Duddos Stones, ancient standing stones, at the top of a field with an amazing panoramic view. Standing stones are something I have always been fascinated by, and it was great to go there and absorb their energies.

I soon found out that I had a lot to learn about living in a caravan. It was certainly a new way of life and I found myself being very grateful for the smallest of things that before I had just taken for granted. I immersed myself into caravan living. The caravan was just going to be a base, a where we could store our stuff and live between travelling to different places.

One thing that I did from the day I left Helensburgh was keep a diary of all the different places that I visited. This is great for me now to remember exactly what I've done, and it will be something that I will always keep.

The first thing that we did was prepare ourselves to walk the Berwick Coastal Route and the Northumberland Coastal Route. We did these walks in stages, covering between 18km and 30km in a day, but not walking on consecutive days. The two routes combined were a total of 145km/90 miles - from Scotland over the border to England, down the east coast of the United Kingdom. For most of it you are walking alongside the North Sea. The views are stunning, with lots of different terrains. We did the last stage in two consecutive days; from Bamburgh to Almouth the first day, which was 35km and from Almouth to Cresswell the following day, which was 26km. That was tough. The first day, we walked a bit more than my feet could handle. I had blisters and at one point felt a searing pain in both my pinkie toes. I'm not quite sure how I managed the second day, but I limped the whole way determined that I was going to finish it. A couple of weeks later, I lost both toenails on my pinkie toes. Thankfully, they have now grown back. It was a wonderful achievement and it didn't put me off every a walk like this again. I loved every moment of it.

On 11th May, we travelled to Richmond and stayed there for a couple of days, enjoying the area's beauty. We then travelled to Keswick in the Lake District, where we attended a hypnotherapy weekend. This event made me fall in love with hypnotherapy, and later in the year, I signed up to train as a hypnotherapist. I did my six-month training with the Jacquin Academy. This is a father and son team. They are the perfect teachers, both teaching in their own way and bringing a different perspective. They have similar but different styles; they work as a team and treat everyone like family, and they are both truly inspirational. This course not only gives you the skills to become a hypnotherapist, but is also very healing. You get to meet people from all over the world and practise with them, allowing you to let go of any issues you may have, and everyone is keen to help each other. Doing this course allowed me to get over my fear of using video communications for work and helped me gain confidence, not only in myself, but to set up my new business online.

On 20th May, we flew to Paphos in Cyprus, where we were spending the next month. Oh, I love Cyprus! Waking to sunshine every day is definitely good for the soul. Every morning, we would go for a run, normally around 5km, and then swim - initially in the pool where we were staying, but eventually in the sea. Swimming in the sea has always been a fear of mine so this was another achievement. Not only did I let go of my fear of swimming in the sea, I grew to love it and would crave it. We did a lot of sightseeing too. We hired bikes and we walked lots and just enjoyed every moment. The month went by very quickly.

We came back from Cyprus and I came to Helensburgh for a few days. Although I loved being away, I also missed my family a lot. I did find it hard, being use to seeing them most days. So throughout my time away, I would come back to Helensburgh for a few days or a long weekend every few weeks. After coming back from Helensburgh this time, I met with my friend and we went to Brighton for a week, staying at the same hotel as we had the previous year. We did lots of sightseeing, ate lots of nice food and danced the days away outside our hotel.

I came back from Brighton and we began looking for a new camper van. It took us until the 18th August to find the right van for us, and we named him Bertie. Before getting Bertie, we explored Berwick upon Tweed, Durham, Helensburgh, Richmond and Bulgaria. I had never been to Bulgaria before and would go back again. This was a proper beach holiday for us. We sunbathed, swam, went for massages and even danced at an afternoon foam party - another first, that was so much fun. We drove to Southport when we came back from Bulgaria and spent a weekend there with my family, celebrating my sister's big birthday.

It was so exciting when we picked up Bertie, from Teeside on 6th September. The first place we went was Scarborough. Waking up in Bertie overlooking the North Sea was a great experience. We then travelled to Skipsy, Filey, Whitby, Seaham, Durham, Haswell, Haltwhistle, Longtown, Annan, Girvan, Irvine and Balloch, where my grandsons stayed overnight with us. They found this so exciting and loved sleeping over in Bertie. We stayed in lots of different campsites and also did a bit of wild camping. Unfortunately, three days after setting off in Bertie we had an accident in him. No-one was hurt and we could still travel in him, but it did end up in months of frustration waiting on the repairs getting done. It would take nine months in total to get this all sorted.

On 29th September, we travelled to Helensburgh for a couple of days to meet up with family. Then on 1st October, we went to Glasgow and did the Great North Run. This was my second 10k, and it felt as good as it did the first time. The rest of October was spent a lot in Berwick, where I was studying hypnotherapy and creating my new business.

On 11th November, we flew to Gibraltar. I had never been to Gibraltar before; another place I would recommend and will go back to one day. Gibraltar was fun. We met lots of nice people and walked the Gibraltar Rock. I'm not sure if I would go back there though, as I had a scary experience. We were at the top of Gibraltar Rock, with hundreds of tourists around. I was standing, minding my own business, when one of the big macaques monkeys, jumped on my back. He had one hand scratching around my face and one hand trying to open my rucksack. I don't think I've ever been so scared when this ton weight jumped on top of my back and neck. I heard myself scream, and then I stood motionless, too petrified to move, until my partner came and got him off. As we walked away, I noticed everyone was pointing and staring, and I just wanted to get away from them all. I found myself scared the whole way down, and I was shaking every time I had to pass the many macaques on the track.

We spent a great weekend in Gibraltar before walking over the border to La Linea, Spain and spending 10 days there. It was good to see Spain out of holiday season, but we did return to Gibraltar often. We came back to the UK on the 25th November.

December wasn't the best month and cracks began to appear in the relationship. I spent the first week of the month in Helensburgh, then went back to Berwick. It was below freezing the second week of that December and the caravan was cold. The water froze, the boiler broke and the waste frozen. We ended up staying in different hotels near Newcastle. I came back to Helensburgh for Christmas and New Year and took unwell again; my body was getting all the symptoms of M.E. My body was telling me that things weren't right. I was going to have to make changes again!!!

I love travelling and seeing different places and it was a good way for me to rediscover my likes and dislikes. I also faced a lot of my fears whilst away. If you want to rediscover who you are, you have to face your fears. Over the years, every time I feel that feeling of fear in my chest or stomach - that feeling of tightness and nausea - I know that to grow as an individual, I have to face that fear. This feeling is so familiar to me now that I push myself to the limit to face it head-on. I get to grips with every sensation - every feeling - and find a way to overcome it. It is not easy, in fact it is extremely difficult, but I don't want to live with any regrets. I ask myself "In five years' time, will you look back with regret that I didn't do this?" The answer for me is normally always "Yes" and I do not want to live this precious life with any regrets.

Live your life with no regrets. You will be so amazed at what you can achieve when you do this!!

I came back to Berwick-upon-Tweed at the beginning of January and for a week I didn't get any better. In fact my health was deteriorating and I knew I had to make big changes yet again so that my body would be back in balance. So I made the difficult decision to leave Berwick 1 and leave my partner. I found myself homeless and having to start all over again. Deep down though, I knew everything would be alright. Everything would work out; it always does. It's just another step on the path, another fear to face.

THE COURAGE TO BEGIN AGAIN AFFIRMATIONS/MANTRAS

- I have the strength to rebuild my life in new and beautiful ways.
- Every ending is an opening to something greater.
- I trust the unknown and step forward with courage.
- I am free to create a life that reflects my soul.
- Starting over is a gift I give myself.

EMPOWERING HEALING SUGGESTIONS/TECHNIQUES

1. RELEASE & WELCOME RITUAL - Write down one thing you are letting go of and one thing you are inviting in. Burn the first, keep the second somewhere visible.
2. TRAVEL AS MEDICINE - Visit a new place, even locally to awaken fresh perspectives.
3. LIGHTNESS INVENTORY - Go through one area of your home and clear out items that no longer feel aligned.
4. DAILY POSSIBILITY PROMPT - Ask yourself each morning: "What's one small thing I can do today to create a better tomorrow?"
5. ANCHOR IN GRATITUDE - Before bed, write down three ways you felt supported by life that day.

JOURNALING REFLECTION QUESTIONS

- What will I gain by letting go of my old life?

- How does travel or time away shape my perspective?

- What fears will I face by starting over again?

- How would I want my "new chapter" to feel?

- What symbols or signs remind me I am on the right path?

- Additional reflection or memories that surface.

THE PHOENIX WITHIN

There is a fire that does not destroy -
It transforms.
You stood in the ashes
Of the life you once knew,
The smoke still curling around your feet.

It hurt to let go.
It hurt to stand there,
Not knowing who you would become.

But slowly, the embers began to glow,
Not from the world outside,
But from within you.

You rose - not in a rush,
But with steady, certain steps.
Each day, a new feather of courage.
Each breath, a reminder that you were born for this.

The world was not ending - it was beginning again,
Though you.

And as you walked forward, higher, freer, you knew the truth.
The phoenix was never a myth.
It was always inside you, waiting for you to remember.

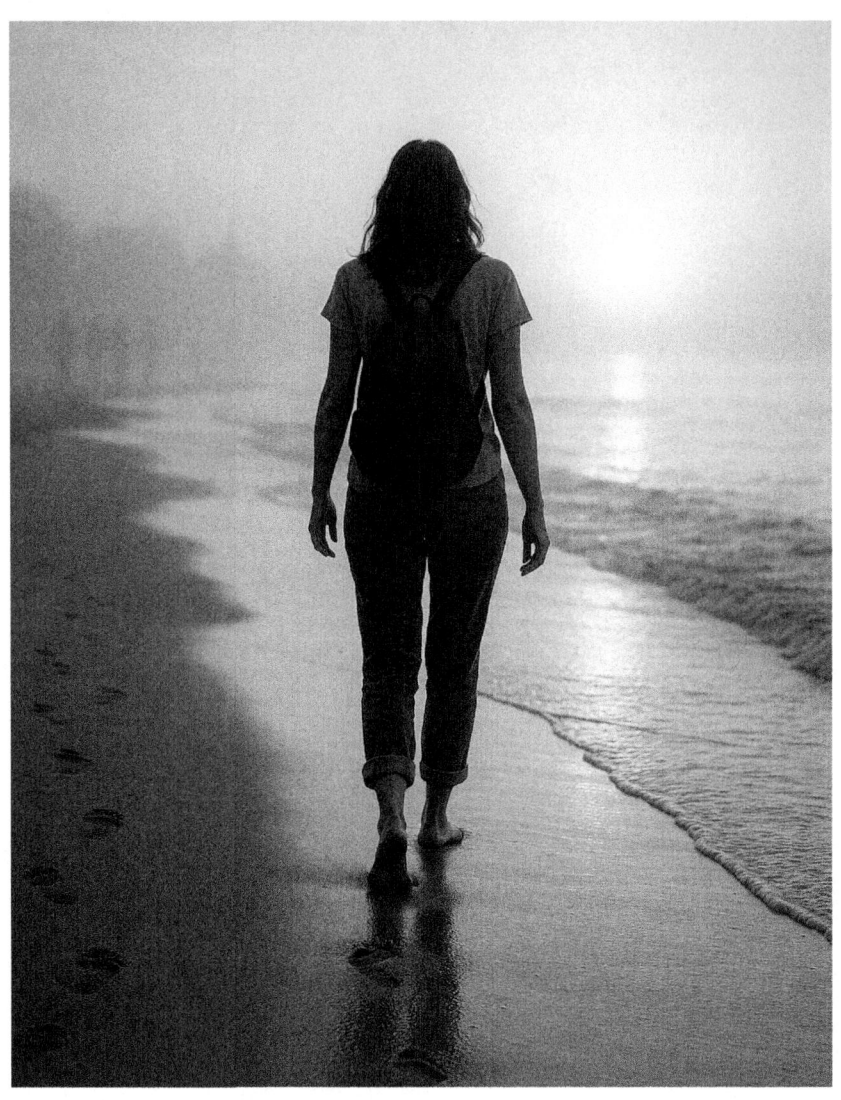
The Courage to Begin Again

CHAPTER 8 - HOMELESS

On 28th January 2023, I packed my car with all my belongings from the caravan in Berwick-upon-Tweed. What was I going to do now that I had made this decision? I had no home, just a few belongings and a car. I headed for Scotland and booked into a Bed and Breakfast in a tiny village called Athlestaford on the east coast, in the middle of nowhere, so I could have some time to think about my next steps, and to start healing my body again. The one thing I've noticed over the years is that anytime I become unwell it's normally when my life isn't balanced and I have to make some big changes.

Whilst staying at Athlestaford, I did a lot of soul-searching. I meditated, journaled and went on long walks. I spoke to my family to let them know what was happening, and to let them know I was OK. My sister, kindly said I could stay in her spare bedroom until I found somewhere to live - something that I'm truly grateful for. After a few days at the B&B, I made my way to Balloch and settled into my sister's home.

I took me a good bit of time to start feeling better again. I think the stress of those weeks had taken its toll on me, but I came to the decision to do some more travelling - this time on my own. I would then find somewhere to live and start working again in my hometown, bringing with me the new skills that I had learnt over the last year. I knew I had changed, but the next couple of months would see me change and grow more into my authentic self.

Over the next few weeks, I did a lot of healing, walking and meeting up with with family and friends. I decided I had to get away somewhere and do a bit of travelling myself. It was the middle of winter and I didn't want too go to far for my first adventure, so I booked a coach trip away for a weekend in Blackpool.

On 25th February, I got a train to Glasgow, went to Buchanan bus station and boarded the coach for Blackpool. I was a little nervous about doing this myself, but I also felt proud of myself as this was another hurdle that I was about to jump. I settled on the coach, listened to some music on my earphones and enjoyed the journey. We had a tea break stop halfway through the journey, at Gretna Green. As I got off the coach, I noticed everyone else seemed to be in couples or groups, but again I said to myself, "I've got this. Just enjoy". I got myself a coffee and then walked around. When we arrived in Blackpool, the coach dropped people off at different hotels. Mine was the last stop. I got off the coach, checked in and went to my room. I unpacked my small suitcase and went for a walk along the Blackpool promenade.

Dinner was at 5 p.m., so I went to my room got showered and ready, and went down for dinner. I was really nervous at this point, walking into the dining room on my own and sitting in the restaurant on my own. I was determined though; nothing was going to stop me, not even that queasy feeling in my stomach. I was the only person on my own, but to be honest I got on alright and people-watched as I ate my dinner. Later on that evening, I went down to the entertainment myself. I knew this was another fear that I had to face. The entertainment kept choosing me to play the games and at the end of it, I just thought. "Why not?" I could just relax and enjoy and this it so, this is what I did. When the music came on, people got me up to dance and I got chatting to others. What I noticed was that when you're on your own, people do tend to make more of an effort to include you, and it wasn't as bad as my fears had lead me to believe.

Next morning at breakfast, people were all saying hello. I then went another walk along the promenade. On the way back I went to visit one of the gypsy fortune tellers. Again, I thought, "Why not?" As soon as I sat in her booth she told me she could feel all the spiritual energies coming off me. She asked, if this was the type of work I did. I laughed and said I did readings too and proceeded to give her a reading as well. In the evening when I went for dinner, sitting alone did not bother me at all. I skipped the entertainment as I was feeling tired and instead just had an early night. Next morning, I had breakfast, packed my case and went for a walk before the bus picked everyone up again to head back to Glasgow. The journey went well, stopping for a break did not bother me this time, and I went to a cafe and had something to eat. I got back to Glasgow safely, boarded the train back to Dumbarton then picked up my car and headed back to my sister's.

I had done it. I had gone away for the weekend solo on a coach tour and even turned my fear of doing this into something I had enjoyed and grown from. I was now ready to take the next step and book an overseas trip by myself. This was something I did the very next day, I booked myself on a week-long yoga retreat in Spain.

On 18th March, I drove to Edinburgh Airport, parked my car and got on a plane to Malaga, Spain. Travelling by myself and going to somewhere new did not bother me this time. In fact, I was excited. When I reached Malaga, the lady running the course picked me up, then picked another lady up from the bus station in Malaga and we headed to Calahonda where the retreat was being held. I was shown to my room, which was fantastic. I had the top floor to myself with an en-suite bedroom and a very large balcony with beautiful views.

That week was one of the best weeks I've ever had and I made some lovely friends. There were five of us in total. The couple hosting the retreat were from Italy, and there was a lady from England, a lady from Portugal and myself. We ate together, did yoga on the beach every morning and went out on day trips. We all bonded so well together and the week was spent having lots of fun and laughter. I am still in touch with them all.

One of those days spent there will forever be etched on my mind. I will never forget it. I am definitely a hippie at heart and have always wanted to go to a hippie camp and experience it and soak up the atmosphere. And this was what I got to do.

The lady from Portugal was staying at a hippie camp, situated on a large block of rented land, where the residents grew their own fruit and vegetables and lived off the land. When I found out about the camp's ceremony to celebrate the spring solstice. I got this growing feeling of excitement and asked if we could go. And we could. We did "Biodanza", dancing, drumming, singing and other activities, and it was just magical. I felt so alive and everyone was so nice; you could feel the love and happiness that radiated from them. I loved every moment of it. I didn't sleep much that night as I was reliving everything that had happened. The next day we laughed the whole day, not just a giggle but big belly laughs. The energy that radiated from us was fantastic.

During my stay at the yoga retreat, I told my yoga teacher that I was considering doing yoga teacher training. This is something I had been thinking about for a long time, as I wanted to run wellness workshops and felt this was something that would make my workshops complete, along with other skills that I had. I got a recommendation for a yoga teacher that did the training in Marbella, and I booked myself on a three-week course that started on the 2nd May.

The week at the retreat, went so quickly, even though we had packed so much in. We had all grown very close, very quickly and I think everyone felt sadness when it was time to say our goodbyes. I sat at Malaga airport waiting for my plane and it crossed my mind that I really had to find my own home again. As I sat in the airport I prayed to the angels. "Please help me find my perfect new home quickly". That's exactly what they did and within three weeks in was living in my new home.

I began looking for and viewing places to stay, on 10th April, I kept intuitively getting the name of a lady that I knew had moved to a caravan park the year before. I had been toying with the idea of living in a caravan, so I contacted her to ask her how she found caravan life and to get some information from her. During our conversation, she gave me the telephone number of a lady who had the keys to a residential park home around the peninsula, which was around a half-hour drive from Helensburgh. I contacted the lady and before I knew it, I was meeting her a couple of hours later to view the property.

I hadn't realised that this caravan park had residential park homes, but when I saw it, I just knew it was the right place for me. The lady that took me around the house also showed me around the park and gave me lots of information and the telephone number of the lady selling it. I drove back to my sister's knowing that this was the right move, but before I made any commitment, I phoned my children to see what they thought. They thought it sounded perfect for me. I gave myself that night that sleep on it. I awoke the next morning and phoned the lady selling it. One week later on 17th April, I had the keys to my new home.

It needed quite a bit of work doing. I started the very next day and then three days after getting the keys, I moved in. I had to start all over yet again, but this didn't bother me. I loved organising my new things, as well as all the organising and preparing my new colour schemes. This kept me really busy. In the middle of all this I had my yoga teacher training course to go to - talk about everything all happening at once.

On 2nd May, I drove to Glasgow airport, parked my car and waited for the plane to go to Malaga airport again. I waited and waited, but the plane kept being delayed. Finally, it was confirmed the plane was cancelled. Oh no, my course was starting the very next morning and now I couldn't be there in time. There was quite a commotion at the airport as people began to panic and get irritated that the plane had been cancelled. I remained calm and just thought, "Ah well, where will this adventure take me now?". Eventually, after several hours of waiting and not being sure of what was happening, everyone got put up in hotels in Glasgow and told that there was a plane being was scheduled to take us the next afternoon. We were all taken to the hotel in taxis. I contacted the yoga teacher and explained what was happening and that I would be there, but I would be a day late. I do not like being late for anything and always strive to be early, but I had no choice but to surrender to it. This wasn't an easy thing for me to do, but I did. The normal thoughts and fears did start to creep in, uncertainly about turning up a day late knowing that everyone in the class had already had a day to start bonding. I couldn't allow myself to become out of balance with my fears so I began meditating and stating positive affirmations, confirming that everything would work out and that I had nothing to worry about.

I did manage to get a few hours of sleep at the hotel. We were provided with our breakfast in the morning before getting picked up by a taxi and taken back to the airport. Again, I had been thrown out my comfort zone, but had met some lovely people in the process of and everything did work out; it always does. Arriving at the airport felt like deja vu. I went through the exact same process as the previous day, but this time the plane left on time.

I arrived at Malaga airport in the late afternoon, to find I was no longer able to get picked up by car to get taken to the accommodation, as would have happened the day before. I now had to get public transport to the Marbella bus station, which was about an hour away, and would get picked up there. Another fear I would have to face as I had never done this before, in a country where I didn't speak the language. I shouldn't have worried though; it did work out and I did manage OK. I asked a couple of people that had been on my plane how to get a bus to Marbella and they told me I had to go to the bus station, which was just outside the airport, and purchase a ticket there. I'm so grateful that they gave me this information, and I found the whole process of booking the bus and getting onboard fairly easy. I had to wait just under two hours for the bus, as the first one to arrive was fully booked, but I did get the bus and I did get to Marbella myself. Yes I was all happy with myself! This was another achievement for me, helping me grow in confidence.

I got picked up from Marbella bus station by the yoga teacher and taken to La Cala de Mijas, where the training was taking place. I got there around 10 p.m. Finally, I was at the teacher training course. There were another three girls on the course. They were all from Germany, but had come separately. They came to welcome me when I arrived. How things had changed from all those years ago, when I was so nervous and unable to talk to anyone. Here I was walking into a house in a different country, meeting strangers that I was about to spend the next three weeks studying with and I wasn't nervous. I was excited for all the experiences that were ahead.

Early next morning, we began our training. I loved this course, this experience, and the class bonded well, which was a good job as we were all living together and spending most of our waking hours together. We did a lot of practical work as well as theory, and at the end bought everything into practise to run our own class. We had one afternoon/evening off during that time, and I arranged to meet the yoga teacher and her husband who had hosted the retreat I went to in March. I was so pleased with myself as I set off to Malaga. The other girls had helped me plan my journey - I had to get a bus to Fuengorola , then a train to Malaga. I travelled there myself. I had even been offered a lift to Malaga by one of the girls who was going there for the day, but I explained that getting public transport was something I had to do for myself, another hurdle I wanted to cross. She understood, and we met up later in Malaga to travel back to our accommodation together. I felt proud of myself. It had been a lovely day and I had enjoyed meeting friends and achieving my new goals.

The time went quickly and I came back from Spain, not only a yoga teacher, but feeling amazing, mentally, physically, emotionally and spiritually. We trained in a lot of different types of yoga. Most mornings saw us practise on the beach. We were living the dream. I loved the training and I was excited to share my new skillset with others.

Sitting at Malaga airport awaiting my return flight was a different experience than it had been two months before. Everything had changed; I had my new home to return to, I was excited about returning to work, and I was feeling great and really optimistic - a new person from compared to when I had first taken this time off.

I came back from Spain and continued doing the work that needed doing in my new home. I loved it at the caravan park. The drive from the airport had been exciting; as I was so grateful to have my new home. I enjoyed doing the work and it didn't take too long for things to start to take shape.

On 3rd July, I went away again, this time to Corfu and I wasn't alone - my sister and my niece came with me. This was my first-ever girls' holiday overseas; another new experience. The hotel was beautiful and had only been opened a month, and the staff were really friendly. We arrived at the hotel at 11pm, just as the Greek night they were hosting was finishing. We had to join the circle, for the last dance, smashing plates as they do in the Greek tradition, before we were taken to our rooms. What a way to start a holiday! I knew this was going to be a great week, and it was: lots of sunshine, sunbathing, reading, eating good food and enjoying the town's many tribute bands, where we danced and sang along. We had a lot of laughs and a fantastic week in Corfu and I thought, "I'm so happy."

When we came back, it was my son's 21st birthday party. Where had all the years gone? It was quite a nostalgic time for me as I remembered when he was born and

I hardly had the energy to get through the day, and now I danced the night away. So much in my life had changed.

On 3rd August, I went to Brighton with my friend for a long weekend. This was our third year in a row. We had a great time there. The weekend coincided with the annual pride weekend, and although the weather wasn't great that year we had our usual laughs and danced away and had the bonus of watching the parade. My niece and some of her friends joined us for a couple of days and we had such a good time.

At the start of the year, I found myself homeless. But so much had happened since and everything had worked out. I would say this to anyone wishing to make changes but scared of what the outcome will be. Trust and believe! Face the fear and believe that everything will work out. Unless you take steps towards your happiness you will never know how it will work out. I like to say, "What if?". What if, taking that step, trusting and believing, will make you so much happier. The universe has your back. You just have to overcome the fear that is standing in your way.

Trust and believe!!

After I came back from Brighton, and having had time for a lot of reflection on which direction my life was going and who I was, I came to another decision with an important realisation: I had now become the authentic ME

UNSHAKEABLE SPIRIT AFFIRMATIONS/MANTRAS

- I am safe, even in uncertain places.
- My worth is not defined by my circumstances.
- Every step forward is proof of my strength.
- I trust myself to find the way through.
- I carry my home with me.

EMPOWERING HEALING SUGGESTIONS/TECHNIQUES

1. ANCHOR OBJECT - Keep a small object (stone, crystal, or talisman) with you as a reminder of your inner strength.
2. RESOURCE GRATITUDE -Each day , write down one person, skill, or resource that is helping you right now.
3. DAILY GROUNDING PRACTICE - Stand tall, feet on the ground, breathe deeply, and affirm, "I am rooted, I am unshakable."
4. MICRO-MOMENTS OF JOY - Seek out small pleasures - a warm drink, a sunrise - as nourishment for the spirit.
5. REFRAME THE STORY - Instead of "I am lost," affirm, "I am between chapters, on the way to my next home>"

JOURNALING REFLECTION QUESTIONS

- How did I discover strength I didn't know during a difficult time?

- What does "home" mean to me beyond a physical space?

- Who or what helped me when I had little?

- How did I keep hope alive in moments of fear or uncertainty?

- What part of me will never be the same after this experience?

- Additional reflection or memories that surface.

THE ROAD STILL RISES

They could take the walls, the roof,
The keys in your hand -
But they could not take you.

You walked through the nights,
Colder than your bones had known,
And mornings where the air felt heavy with doubt.

Still, your feet kept moving,
Still, your heart refused to close.

You found that "home"
Was not made of bricks or beams -
It was stitched into your breath,
Your laughter,
The way you spoke your name with pride.

And even as the road stretched on,
You carried something unbreakable.

Some would call it resilience.
Some would call it faith.
But you know -
It is the fire of your spirit, and it will light your way
Until the doors open again.

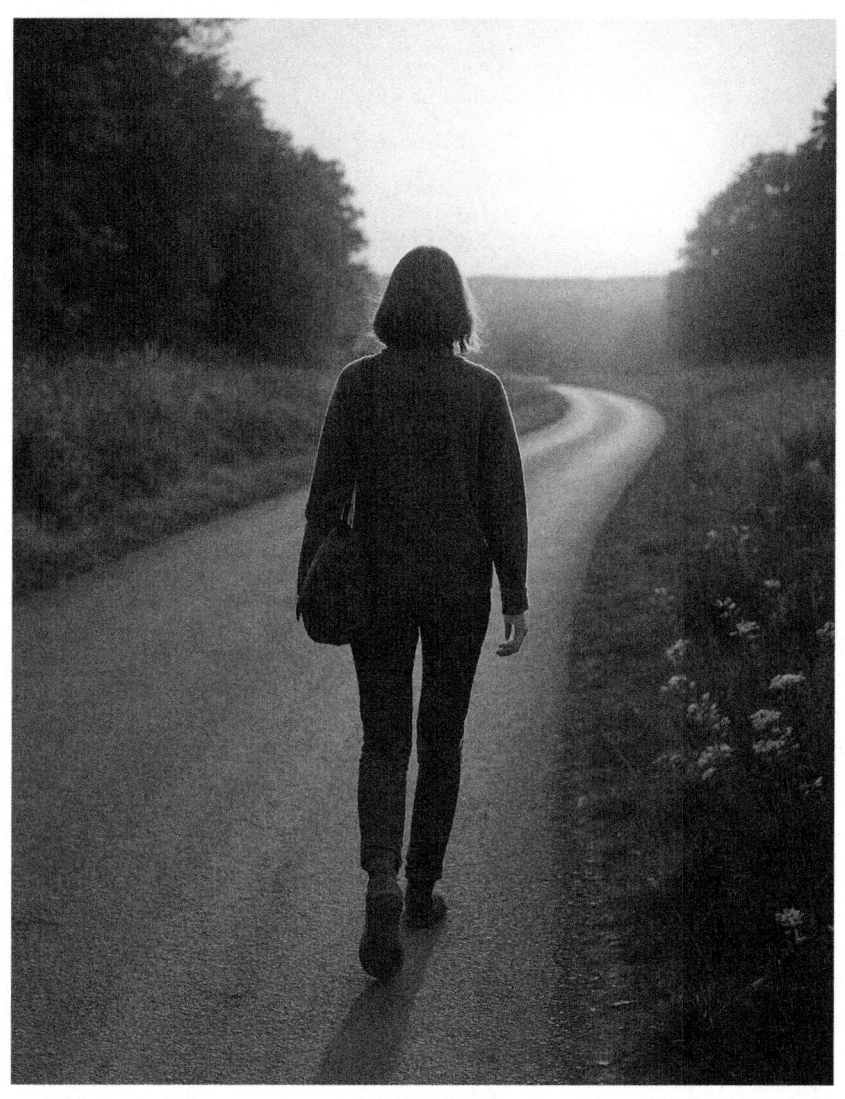

Unshakeable Spirit

CHAPTER 9 - THE DISCOVERY

In 1998, I became so unwell and I had no idea how much this would change my life. When I look back now 25 years has gone past so quickly, and so much has happened. There were times I felt such despair. I couldn't understand why I had become so unwell and I couldn't see a way out. I look at that illness as a gift now. It is something I will always have to live with, but it has taught me so many life lessons and much about myself and what I am actually capable of. If you had told me then what I know now, I'm not sure that I would have believed you.

I was living a life where I was overworking, overstressed and unhealthy, mentally, physically, emotionally and spiritually. I didn't realise this at the time, and it wasn't a quick fix to get to where I am now. It has taken of lot of learning and understanding to change myself. It has been a long process, but strangely enough the time has gone by in a blink of the eye. Writing this has given me a new understanding of how much I have learnt and how far I have come.

Through strength and determination, I have faced many fears and made so many discoveries. I love life and this year I decided to do something that I have never done before. I have decided to give myself something that I have only given to others and not to myself - unconditional love.

For all these years, I didn't know who I was and what I wanted. Ever since I was a little girl, it has always bothered me that I didn't fit in. I have never felt that I fitted in, but now I don't want to fit in. I am who I am, and I love myself for who I am.

Although I haven't got everything sussed out, and I'm certainly not perfect in any way, I do realise that life has so much to teach us. I understand that I have so much more to learn and so many fears that I will have to face. But I also know that many more opportunities that will be presented to me along the way.

Life is short, and we have to make the most of it. We have to grab every opportunity and be totally true to ourselves. We have to live with love in our hearts, rather than fear, and we have to understand this to be able to grow in all areas of our lives.

Life is full of lessons that we can either grow from or be stuck with repeating the same loop. To grow we have to take that step. We also have to face that fear and sometimes it is really scary, but when you do and you look back, you must remember to congratulate yourself for your achievements. All too often, we don't take time to look at how far we have come and all the challenges and obstacles we have faced. Sometimes, or maybe a lot of times, we don't give ourselves the credit we deserve. We have to give ourselves kindness and respect. Nobody gives us a manual at the start of our lives; we are here to learn and grow.

Giving ourselves love and understanding ourselves is a big step in making changes. We must be grateful for what we have. If we are grateful, we can make these changes. If we live in fear, we get stuck, we can't see a way out, and we have to change this to be able to move forward. The more we love, the more gratitude we have for everything, the more strength and determination we have to make more positive changes in our life. This is how we begin to change and grow as a person. The first thought in our head, when we wake up in the morning should be a big thank you for being alive and having another day to live. Then we should begin making plans for it to be the best day possible. We have to choose to have control over our lives, instead of our lives having control over us. We must begin to make our own choices and then live by them.

I had lived my life for everyone else and worried about others' expectations and opinions of me. I wasn't being true to myself or living my authentic life. I didn't realise all those years ago how important it was to look after yourself, mind, body and soul. This story is about living, understanding and growing from M.E. It is a story about M.E. but it is also a story of finding ME.

It felt important and right for me to share this story in the hope that it can help someone. Life can be difficult for us, although I now believe it is how we look at it that helps us in how we deal with it and in turn how it makes us feel. I know that it isn't always perfect - all rainbows and unicorns - but allowing ourselves the gift of understanding ourselves and changing our emotions will, in turn, make us more able to make a big difference. I certainly still have to give myself a good talking to now and again and sometimes up the practises I have put in place in my life to get myself back into balance. I now know my triggers. I'm able to understand myself so much more than I ever did. I am still learning though, and will eternally be doing so.

Having had the experience of not being well enough to do anything, I definitely make the most of every moment of life to the best of my ability. As I write this, I am again making many more changes - I have lots of ideas and plans that I wish to implement in my work I want to help others live their life to the best of their abilities and see how making changes in how they live their life on a mental, emotional, physical and spiritual level can bring joy, fulfilment and love.

I end my story with a chapter full of what I have learned over the years to bring about the changes I needed to make a difference to my life. Putting these practises into place will bring forth changes in you, mind, body and soul allowing you to discover more about you and to live your life as the more authentic you.

Healing is not about becoming someone new. It's about remembering who you've been all along.

STANDING IN MY STRENGTH AFFIRMATIONS/MANTRAS

- I honour the journey that shaped me.
- My courage has carried me farther than I ever dreamed.
- I am proud of who I have become.
- Strength is my nature, resilience is my birthright.
- I walk forward with gratitude for every step behind me.

EMPOWERING HEALING SUGGESTION/TECHNIQUES

1. VICTORY JOURNAL - Write down the challenges you've overcome and the strengths you used to do so.
2. MIRROR GRATITUDE - Look into your eyes in the mirror and thank yourself for surviving and thriving.
3. SYMBOL OF STRENGTH - Wear or carry a piece of jewellery, stone or charm that represents your courage.
4. CELEBRATE MILESTONES - Create rituals to honour your personal wins, no matter how small.
5. TEACH FROM EXPERIENCE - Share part of your story with someone who needs hope right now.

JOURNALING REFLECTION QUESTIONS

- What is the greatest lesson my journey has taught me?

- Which moments tested me most, and how did I overcome them?

- How has my definition of "strength" evolved?

- What parts of me am I most proud of today?

- How can I use my strength to help others?

- Additional reflection or memories that surface.

I SEE ME NOW

I see me now -
The person who walked through fire
And came out carrying light.

I am not the same one who began this road,
Head bowed, heart weary,
Searching for a way back.

My scars do not speak of defeat -
They sing of survival.
My eyes do not look away -
They hold the horizon steady.

I have learned that courage is not the absence of fear,
But the choice to keep moving
While the fear walks beside you.

And I know, with certainty that can't be shaken,
That every step I took in the dark was leading me here -
To the place where I could stand tall,
Look the world in the eye and say

"I have found myself,
And I'm not leaving you again."

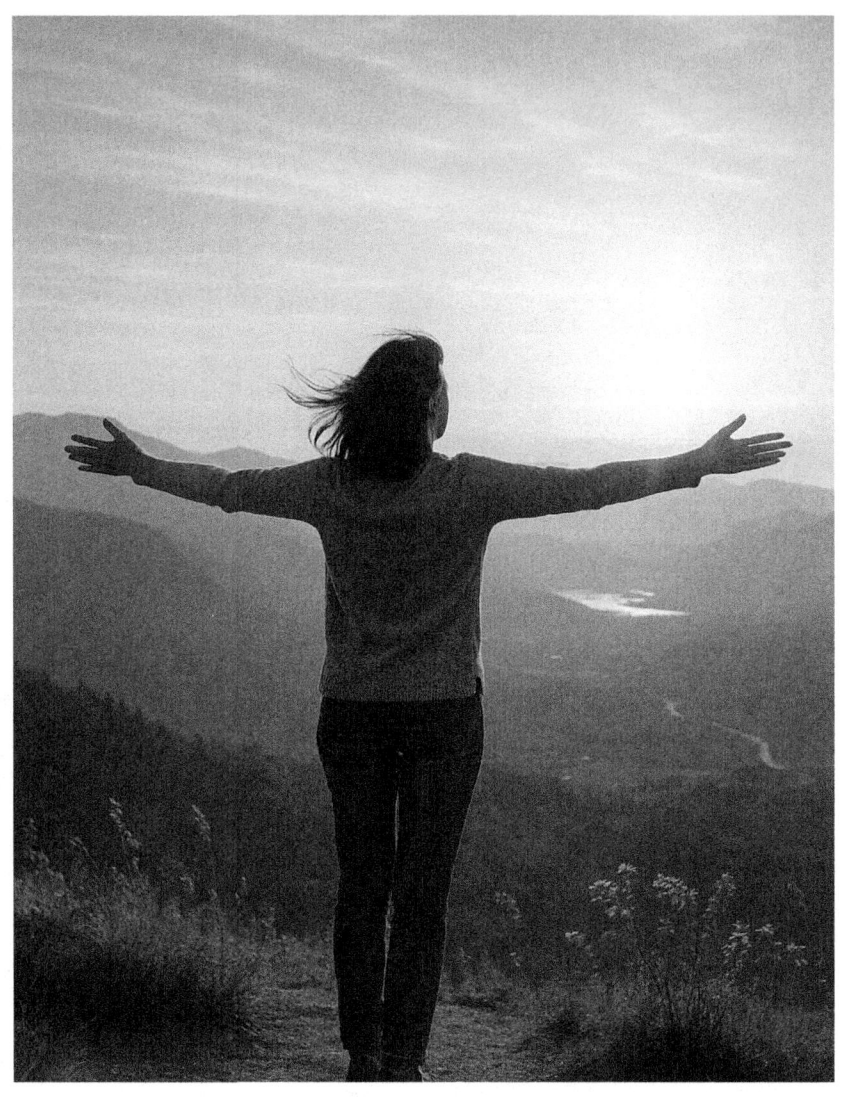
Standing in my Strength

CHAPTER 10 - WHAT I'VE LEARNED IN FINDING ME

Over the last 25 years, I have completely overhauled the way I live my life. Some of these changes took me years to discover and put into practise. These are the practises I have put in place to go from being so unwell with M.E., a condition that left me fatigued and sore and barely leaving my house, to living my life to the full and rediscovering (or maybe finally discovering) ME.

I have found that, in life, it is extremely important for us to have our mind, body and soul completely balanced. I have broken down the lessons I have learned into these three categories and I highly recommend implementing these changes in your life too. You may well be living your life doing some of these important steps, with only a few more changes to make, or you may have to completely overhaul your whole way of living, like I did. What I would suggest is to make one change at a time; don't try to make all the changes at once.

Recognise how well you are doing with every change that you make. Be kind to yourself and be proud of your achievements. Take this one step at a time, and enjoy the process. It takes time for your mind, body and soul to process and integrate these changes; please don't forget that. My hope is that you will learn from what is written here and adjust it as you need to; you have to find out what works well for you. I only want to share what has worked for me, so that it may help you live your life with a new passion and sense of purpose and find out who you are.

MIND

It is important to live in the moment. When we live in fear, we tend to live in the past and when we suffer from anxiety, we tend to live in the future. To be able to live in the moment we have to become aware of our thoughts. A lot of time in life, we live on automatic, so even just being aware of our thoughts can bring many changes.

What we want to be able to do is:

- Let go of fear.

- Let go of anxiety.

- Release negative thoughts.

- Bring in positivity.

- Know what makes us happy.

- Live in the moment.

- Live life with gratitude.

- Have a balanced mind.

- Control our emotions.

- Be able to act, not react.

- Open our minds.

- Speak our truths.

- Celebrate our victories.

The things that I have learned to do to keep my mind in balance are:

- **Meditation -** This is so important and is a learned process. I feel it is about learning what works best for you. Your brain is a muscle, and like any other muscle it takes time and regular practise to grow. Remember this when you start out. There are several different ways to meditate, so experiment with it and find what works best for you. Start off slowly and build your practise; the more you do it, the better you become and you soon begin to notice the benefits. Some different forms of meditation include: focused attention with mindful breathing, guided meditation, repeating mantras, body scans, visualisation, loving kindness meditation (when we send positive energy to ourselves and to others), sound baths and walking meditations.

- **Journaling -** Writing has been a major step in my recovery. It's up to you how you wish to use your journal. You can write about anything. For example, maybe there is something that is worrying you; writing about it and putting it down on paper can help clear your mind. If your mind is full of worry before you go to bed, writing your thoughts and feelings down can help ease and clear your mind so you can get a better night's sleep. You can journal at any time of day, whenever feels right. You can write about your problems. Often putting a problem down on paper or even typing it onto the computer can help you then list potential solutions, easing your mind. You can also journal about your hopes and fears. There is no right or wrong way to journal; it's about doing what feels right for you. You can learn a lot about yourself by journaling and I find that setting the intention and making the time to write can make a big difference. Even if you don't know what to write, just start with that first word and then allow your mind to relax and your hand to write or type - I promise that, the words will begin to flow.

- **Affirmations -** Giving yourself an affirmation for the day changes your mindset. You can choose one that suits you for that day or keep the same one. There are different ways that you can use affirmations; you can say them to yourself all day long or set a timer for every hour to say it. You can say them out aloud if that works better for you or write them setting yourself a set number of times to write them each day. Keep your affirmations positive. A couple of examples of affirmations could be, "I love myself and give myself unconditional love" or "Today is wonderful, good things keep happening to me'. These are just suggestions: use an affirmation or affirmations that suit you.

- **Mindfulness -** I would describe mindfulness as being aware of what is going on in your mind right now. Our mind has a tendency to wander, and unless we are aware of the thoughts that are going around in our head, they tend to just run away with themselves. It is important to be present in the moment and to not be judgemental about our thoughts. This is something that I found difficult at first and what worked for me was repeating the word,"now", it allowed me to come back to the present. The more we become mindful and allow mindfulness to be part of our lives, the more aware we can become of ourselves, allowing changes to our minds and the way that we think. There are different ways that we can practise mindfulness, such as: mindful breathing, body scans, mindful listening, mindful movement, mindful eating and mindful meditation. Mindfulness takes a lot of practise.

- **Intention** - Setting intentions for myself has made such a difference. I set intentions in the mornings for certain things, such as intending to have the best day possible. I set intentions before doing any treatments, for the best possible outcome. I set intentions throughout the day for things to run smoothly. I feel that setting intentions is very important. When manifesting, I set intentions for my goals, dreams and wishes. Setting your intentions throughout the day also allows for big changes within your mind.

BODY

What I've learned about my body is this: the better I treat it, the more respect I give it, the more I look after it, then the better it takes care of me. The four main components of looking after our bodies are: Sleep, Hydration, Exercise and Diet.

- **Sleep** - It is important that you get enough quality sleep every night. Everyone's needs may vary slightly, but adults should generally get between seven and nine hours of sleep each night. Getting can help you:

  o Improve your focus and concentration.

  o Improve your memory.

  o Maintain a healthy weight (with better management of blood sugar).

  o Keep your heart healthy.

  o Keep your immune system strong.

  o Look after your emotional and mental wellbeing.

  o Reduce your stress levels.

  o Keep your circulatory system healthier.

There are different things you can do to help improve your sleep:

o Keep to a regular sleep schedule and wake up at the same time each day - even on weekends. If you have daytime naps, reduce them.

- Increase the daylight your eyes are exposed to, and have an reduce blue light (such as from smartphones, TVs or computers.

- Get some physical exercise during the day.

- Watch what you eat and drink in the evening: don't eat late at night or drink caffeine or too much water.

- Make sure your bedroom is the right environment: cool, clean, uncluttered and relaxing.

- Have a relaxing bath or shower.

- Clear your mind through breath work, meditation or journaling.

- **Hydration** - It is important to drink lots of water throughout the day as your body works so much better if it is well hydrated. It is recommended that you drink at least six to eight glasses of water a day, which is about two litres.

There are many benefits of drinking water, including:

- Replacing fluids, you have lost and through sweating, breathing and going to the toilet.

- Improving digestion and avoiding constipation.

- Helping with circulation.

- Keeping your joints moving.

- Increasing your physical performance.

- Sharpening your focus and concentration.

- Helping you beat tiredness.

- Encouraging you to eat less, (it is common to mistake thirst for hunger).

- Protecting us against disease.

- Prevent dry skin.

Dehydration is serious and can cause headaches, low energy, mental fogginess, moodiness, overeating and/or gaining weight)as it slows down our metabolism), sluggish digestion and fatigue.

- **Exercise -** Physical activity is very important for your body. We should be doing a minimum of 30 minutes a day. I find that it's much easier to exercise when I do something I enjoy. There are still days when I have to give myself a good talking-to, to get started, but I always think about how I will feel after exercising, and I love that feeling so this helps motivate me.

Experiment with it. If you are new to exercise, build it up slowly and find something that you enjoy: it could be walking, swimming, dancing, cycling, yoga, tennis, badminton, football, or doing cardio or weights. Find your passion.

There are ways that you can motivate yourself and stay committed. Try:

- Signing up for a challenge. I've previously signed up for walking challenges through apps, and this always motivates me.

- Signing up to a weekly class.

- Joining a gym or a local swimming pool.

- Arranging to do something with a friend.

- Counting your steps with a fitness tracker: 10,000 a day is recommended.

Do it for you; you are worth it and you will reap the benefits and feel so much better and stronger.

Exercise does so much more for you than you may think.

- It makes you feel happier.

- It can help with weight loss or maintaining a healthy weight.

- It improves muscles strength and is good for your bones.

- It increases your energy levels.

- It can reduce your risk of chronic disease.

- It helps your skin health.

- It is good for your brain health and memory.

- It is good for relaxation and can improve your sleep quality.

- It can help reduce pain.

- It enhances your immune system.

- It gives you a sense of greater wellbeing.

Another thing I would recommend is being outdoors and getting as much daylight as you can. I always feel walking beside water helps cleanse my energy and walking in woods helps to ground me.

- **Diet -** For me, diet makes a massive difference to health. When I changed what I was eating, it did wonders for my health. When we eat the right foods, we give ourselves energy - and so much more. Here is a list of what eating well can do for you:

  - Your body will function better.

- You'll feel more energised.

- You'll begin to crave healthier choices.

- You may experience less inflammation.

- Your gut health will improve.

- Your mood will improve.

- You'll be healthier and stronger.

- You'll have less bloating.

- Your mental focus will increase.

- You will sleep better.

- Your skin will glow more.

- Your metabolism will be faster.

- You may experience lower blood pressure.

You can experiment with different foods to see what agrees with and works for you. I would suggest that you make small changes first. One change at a time will help you work out what works is best for you. Making too many changes at once can put your body into shock. It may help to get some professional help about what foods you should and should not eat. Very briefly, foods to avoid include all processed foods, sugar, white flour products (like bread, biscuits and cakes), highly saturated fats, fast foods and artificial sweeteners. Instead eat more fruit, vegetables, lean proteins, whole grains, beans and pulses.

Changing what you eat will significantly change you in a great way.

Sleep, Hydration, Exercise and Diet are the four aspects of **SHED -** think of shedding the old to bring in the new. Each is essential and they work together: when you start to make changes, one little bit at a time to get them in balance, then you will start to see changes in your body and it will function better.

SOUL

It is important to connect with your soul, and when we do this we can then begin to live our life authentically. I am using the word soul, but I also say my higher self or refer to it as the reiki energy, the universe, the angels, god or goddess. To me, when you connect internally it can be all or one of these words - it's what resonates with you. The important thing is that what we we begin to trust in ourselves and to listen to and tune into ourselves and this has to be done internally. A lot of time in life, we listen to external factors or live our life externally, and this leads us to having an unbalanced life and forgetting how to trust ourselves.

Here are some things I have stopped doing:

- **Listening to other people's opinions** - All too often we listen to what other people say. On most occasions, they do think they are giving the best advice, but honestly just think about it: if you asked 10 people you know well if you should take this new job (maybe its less money but closer to home, or more hours but temporary), I can almost guarantee you would get different advice from every one of them, leading to more turmoil for you. But if you don't look externally and turn within and truly learn to listen to what your internal voice is saying or your gut is telling you, then you will do the right thing.

- **People pleasing** - By this, I mean living your life to suit others. We can all be guilty of putting things off because we are trying to make everyone else happy, but at the end of the day, it is your life and you have to do what makes you happy, it's impossible to please everyone anyway and it is sad that we don't do want we really want to do because of what other people will say or how they will behave. To live authentically, we have to be true to ourselves and live our lives pleasing us, not just pleasing other people. This might sound selfish, but is it? If you are genuinely happy because you are being true to yourself, this happiness will spread to others.

- **Television** - I truly believe that television has too much impact on people's lives, especially if they watch a lot of it. The time you spend watching television is time you are not doing other more fulfilling things and, before you know it hours have gone past. The same can be said for wasting time on our phones and the internet. How easy is it to think I'll just have a quick look at this and the next thing you know an hour has gone by and something you had planned to do has been put off again.

- **News, media, newspapers** - Being involved constantly with what is happening around the world through fear-based stories will leave you with a constant feeling of fear or anxiety. It's impossible to get away from fear if we watch the news a lot. It is a different thing wanting to know what is going on, but fully absorbing ourselves in this and having it going around in our brains, leads us into a vicious circle of engaging with the external world instead of focusing on our internal selves.

I have also learnt that we have to become more aware of our emotions and the effects they are having on us. What are emotions? An emotion is a felt response to something that effects you in some way. It's a mental state associated with thoughts, feelings and behavioural responses.

It's up to us to choose how we feel at any given time.

For example if we have feelings of anger, emptiness, frustration, fear, loneliness, guilt, being misery, loathing or sadness, that has a major impact on our soul, on who we are. There are some things we cannot change, but we can change how we feel about them and we need to become aware of exactly how we feel to be able to make those changes,

This makes awareness so important, and to me this is why we have to become aware and control how we are feeling as often as we can. It is easy to live unconsciously and to carry on each day just existing, unaware of how we are actually feeling. Becoming aware and making a conscious effort to change this will allow massive changes. Everything is energy, and we are all energetic beings. Have you noticed that when you are not feeling good about things, one thing after another goes wrong, whereas if we are feeling good, lots of good things start to happen, lifting your vibration and your emotions. Positive emotions that are good for us include joy, love, gratitude, empowerment, excitement, freedom, happiness, contentment, forgiveness and confidence.

I know that if I allow myself to get stressed, my whole body becomes unwell. This is the time when I increase my practise of all the things that I have listed previously. I know it is the right time for me to make changes. I have to be in control of my emotions to be able to live a normal and fulfilling life.

Here is a list of different things that you can put into practise to help change your vibration and allow yourself to be more in contact with yourself.

- Make time for yourself. Take some timeout to think about what is it that makes you happy, such as a hobby then allow yourself to indulge in this.

- Accept who you are and begin loving yourself. Be aware of your strengths and focus on them; stop putting yourself down.

- Take care of your body. Give your body the attention it needs. It does so much for you, so take great care of it and stop abusing it.

- Practise self-care.

- Do things that makes you feel joyful, enthusiastic, passionate.

- Make someone smile, even when you are passing people in the street or at work, put a big smile on your face and say hello. That can make such a difference to someone else's day and that, in turn, can make such a difference to your day.

- Dance to some uplifting music; it definitely lifts your spirits.

- Declutter. Honestly, how good do you feel once you clear some space. If you have a lot of clutter, don't be overwhelmed by it: write a list of what needs decluttering and tick it off, one step at a time.

- Smell something you love. Spray your favourite perfume or defuse your favourite oils or burn a beautiful scented candle.

- Let go of the past. It's gone and you can't change it, so why hold on to it. Learn from it, grow from it, understand from it.

- Exercise. Find an activity you like and do it. Make it a priority. You will feel so good during it or afterwards.

- Talk a walk in nature or beside water.

- Meditate, either with a guided meditation or some breathing exercises. You could even be just sit and relax to some nice calming music.

- See the good and the positive in everything. Be grateful for what you have and for all the experiences that happen throughout your day.

- Forgive. Don't hold on to resentment or anger, in doing this, you are hurting no-one else but yourself. Try to let go of past hurts.

- Stand up for what you want. If there is something you want, go for it with no regrets. Let go of fear or embrace fear; change your mindset and try to look at that emotion as excitement. Once you have faced that fear, you will feel so pleased with yourself. This helps you to grow and face your next desire or challenge. (One of the mottos that I say to myself is, "In five years time, will I look back and say, I wish I had?" If the answer is yes, the I just do it).

- Express yourself. Be you; don't hold back, don't worry about naysayers and what people are going to say. People always have an opinion, so at the end of the day does it really matter? It might even help others start expressing themselves when they see your confidence in being true to you.

- Do something for someone else. when you do, you brighten up their day and also feel good yourself.

- Read something inspiring or positive. It changes your frequency.

- Journal. You may keep a diary, write your dreams or write your fears. If you have oracle cards, pick one and write down what it says to you. Tuning into a card can help gives you answers, attune to your higher self and trust yourself more.

- Use your intuition: tune into you.

- Eat clean.

- Drink lots of water.

- Be in alignment; be you, love you, enjoy yourself, get to know yourself. What do you like? What's gives you joy and makes you happy? What do you not like? What should you drop that doesn't serve you anymore.

- Do affirmations.

What I have listed in this chapter is what I have learned over the years since becoming unwell at the age of 28. Twenty-five years has gone by quickly, but so much has happened. It hasn't always been easy, and I have made lots of mistakes over the years but by making the changes I have completely changed my life. In fact I am a completely different person to who I was back then.

When I first became ill I couldn't see a way out, but I look now at my illness as a precious gift that has shown me how to lead a more authentic life. In doing so, I have found myself. I know my likes and dislikes and what I want and don't want. It has shown me how to connect my mind, body and soul and I believe that is what we have to do: we have to truly connect everything together and this in turn helps us to live our lives with more balance.

I know I still have a lot to learn, and I am still making mistakes as I go along. When I do make mistakes now, I have learned to laugh at them and look behind that mistake for a lesson that I need to learn. When I do this it helps me to grow spiritually, more and more. I am grateful for life and do see it as a precious gift that we are lucky to be experiencing.

Writing this book has reminded me of all I have been through, and what I have learned. And for all the ups and downs that there has been, I wouldn't change a thing. I have found writing this has been very healing for me, and I hope to help bring healing to others by sharing it.

I would like to say, thank you for taking the time to read my words, and I sincerely hope they help you in some way.

Sending love and healing,

Diane xx

LIVING AS THE WHOLE SELF AFFIRMATIONS/MANTRAS

- My mind is clear, my body is strong, my soul is at peace.
- I live in harmony with my true self.
- Every day, I chose love over fear.
- I honour my mind, body, and spirit equally.

EMPOWERING HEALING SUGGESTIONS/TECHNIQUES

1. MIND-BODY-SOUL CHECK IN - Each morning, ask "What does my mind need today? My body? My soul?" Then honour each answer.
2. ENERGY RESET BREATH - Inhale deeply, imagining fresh light filling you; exhale fully, releasing anything heavy. Repeat three times.
3. JOY LIST - Keep a running list of simple activities that make you happy and do one daily.
4. GRATITUDE & INTENTION PRACTICE - End each day by writing down one thing you're grateful for and one intention for tomorrow.
5. SOUL NOURISHMENT - Set aside weekly time for something purely for your spirit - meditation, nature walks, creative play.

JOURNALING REFLECTION QUESTIONS

- How do I define a "whole and aligned" life for myself?

- What daily habits support my mind, body, and soul?

- What fears have I released to live more authentically?

- How will I continue to nurture my healing in the years to come?

- What is my soul's greatest truth right now?

- Additional reflection or memories that surface.

HOME AT LAST

You have travelled far,
Through storms and stillness,
Through nights you thought would never end,
And mornings that felt like miracles.

You have met yourself in pieces -
The mind searching for answers,
The body longing for rest,
The soul whispering
That you were always whole.

You have learned to listen, too slow down.
To stand tall in the truth of who you are.

No longer chasing, you walk with steady steps,
Knowing that life's not something to survive -
It is something to live.

And here you are, not at he end of the road,
But at the doorway
To everything you have yet to create.

Your heart is light, your spirit is strong,
And your home is not a place -
It is you.

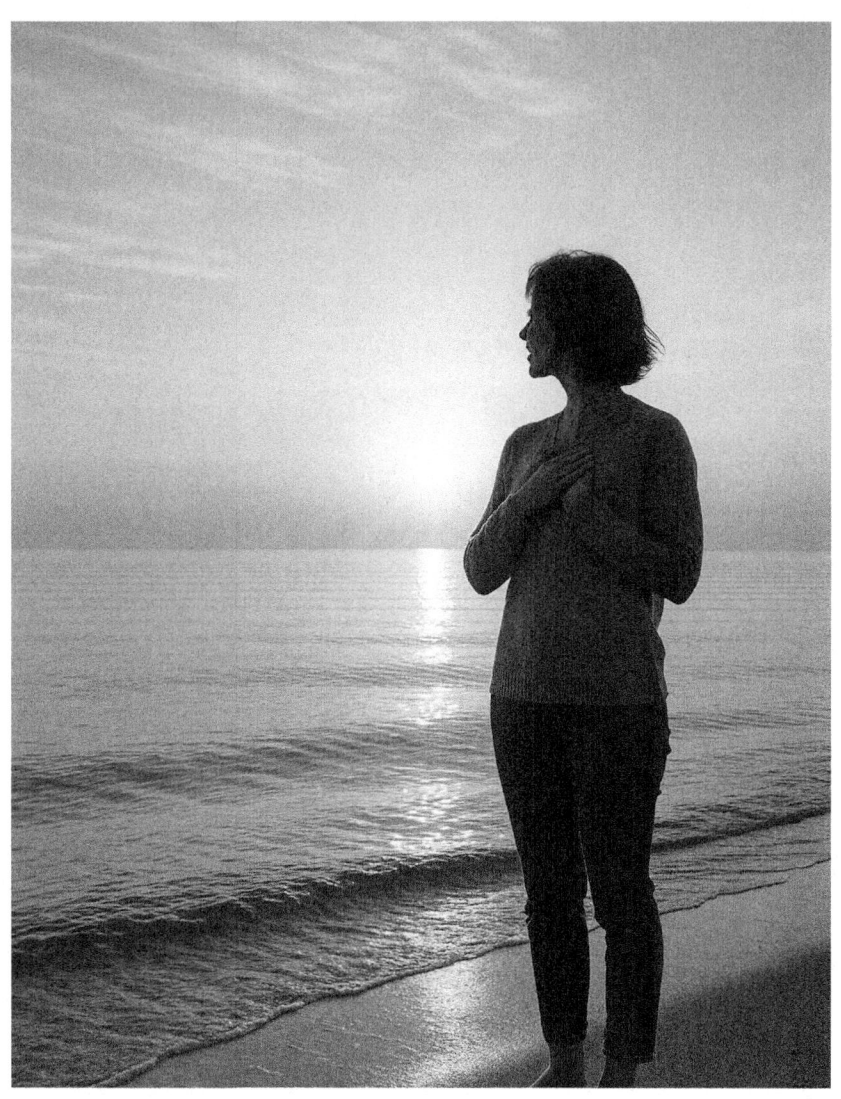

Living as the Whole Self

Dear Reader

Thank you for walking beside me through these pages.
I hope that somewhere within my story, you have found a spark - a word, a moment , a reminder - that speaks to your own heart. My wish is that you feel encouraged to trust your path, to honour your healing, and to believe in the power you hold to create the life you truly desire.

The affirmations and mantras you'll find here are seeds - plant them in your mind and heart, repeat them often, and let them grow into new ways of thinking and feeling. The empowering healing techniques are gentle tools, not tasks; approach then with openness rather than pressure. Let them meet you where you re, and trust that each small step moves you forward.

The journaling prompts are invitations, not obligations. You don't have to have all the answers right away - allow your pen to wander, and you may be surprised by the wisdom that flows within you. These practices are here to be revisited, adapted and carried with you as your journey unfolds.

Life will have its storms, and its sunrises but both will shape you in ways you may not yet understand. Every step, even the ones that feel heavy, can lead you closer to yourself. And in those moments when the way ahead feels unclear, may you ember that you are never truly lost - only in the process of becoming.

A blessing for Your Path

May your heart stay open,
Your steps be steady,
And your spirit remember its strength.
May you meet each day as an unfolding gift,
And may your light - in all its colours -
Shine without fear, without limit, without end.

Wherever life takes you from here, may you walk it with an open heart, knowing you are stronger, wiser, and more radiant than you realise. Our stories are threads in the same tapestry, woven across lifetimes. Until we meet again, you can always find me at www.dianecaroletherapies.co.uk . Id love to ear from you.

Sending love and healing,

Diane Carole

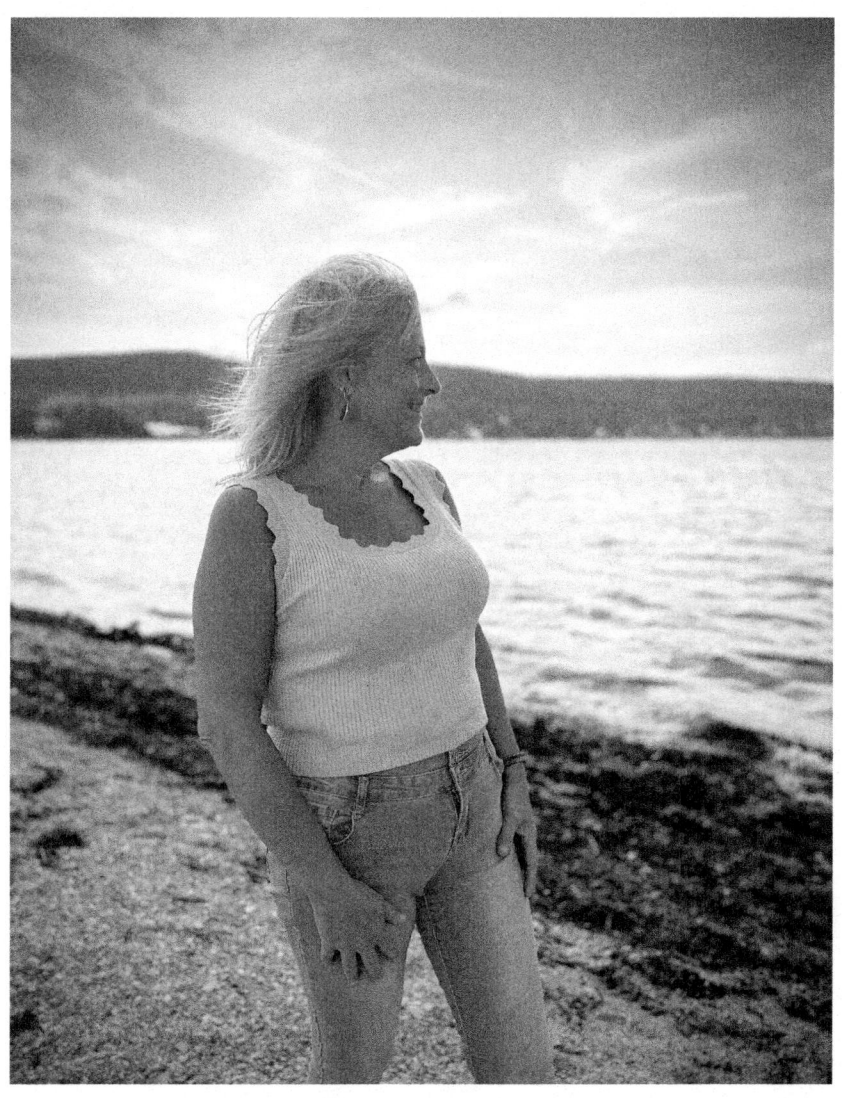

Taken on 15th August 2025
A living reminder that healing is a path walked one step at a time

Printed in Dunstable, United Kingdom